Unlocking Potential: Empowering Adults with Dyslexia

Justin .E Mendez

All rights reserved. Copyright © 2023 Justin .E Mendez

Funny helpful tips:

Stay vigilant about the implications of facial recognition; while powerful, its use raises privacy concerns.

Leverage the potential of augmented reality; it's enhancing user experiences by blending the digital and physical worlds.

*Unlocking Potential: Empowering Adults with Dyslexia :
Breaking Barriers: Unleashing the Hidden Abilities of Adults
Struggling with Dyslexia*

Life advices:

Stay updated with emerging literary genres; they reflect evolving societal interests and concerns.

Practice critical thinking; it helps in making informed decisions.

Introduction

This book appears to be a comprehensive resource that addresses various aspects of dyslexia, its causes, challenges, and management strategies for adults. The guide seems to be well-structured, providing essential information and practical advice for individuals navigating the complexities of dyslexia in their daily lives.

It covers a range of topics, including the key features and common challenges associated with dyslexia, the importance of early intervention, and the process of receiving a diagnosis. The guide emphasizes the need for self-advocacy and effective communication in managing dyslexia, as well as the significance of building a supportive network to help cope with the condition's associated stress.

Moreover, the guide offers strategies to improve literacy skills, including an overview of the Orton-Gillingham approach and practical exercises for enhancing phonological awareness and other literacy-related skills. It also delves into methods for sharpening auditory, visual, and spatial skills, as well as enhancing executive functioning abilities.

Additionally, the guide highlights the inherent strengths associated with dyslexia and encourages readers to embrace these strengths to their advantage. It acknowledges the societal shift toward neurodiversity and the increasing accommodation of diverse learning styles in workplaces and educational institutions. The guide provides practical strategies for building upon these strengths, ultimately helping readers boost their self-confidence and thrive in various aspects of life.

Overall, this book appears to offer valuable insights and guidance for individuals with dyslexia, empowering them to better understand and manage their condition while leveraging their unique strengths to achieve personal and professional success.

Contents

Let's Talk about Dyslexia 1
    What Causes Dyslexia? 3
    Why Is Dyslexia So Misunderstood? 5
    The Key Features of Dyslexia 6
    Processing Difficulties Related to Dyslexia 7
    How Do You Receive a Diagnosis? 9
    The Importance of Early Intervention 9
    The Common Challenges of Dyslexia 11
    Dyslexia Affects Everyone Differently 16
    You Can Successfully Manage Your Dyslexia (But There Is No Cure) 17
    This Book Will Show You How 19
    Conclusion 19

Navigate Dyslexia as an Adult 20
    Common Signs and Struggles 21
    You May Have Been Struggling for Years without Knowing It 24
    Being an Adult Is Hard; Dyslexia Can Make Navigating Adulthood Harder 24
    Everyone Has Their Challenges and Their Gifts 29
    Get Clear on What You Need to Succeed 29
    Remember, You Are Your Best Advocate 31

- Communicate Your Needs 32
- Surround Yourself with a Supportive Team 33
- Make an Action Plan 34
- You Will Always Be Dealing with Dyslexia 35
- It Takes Dedication and Hard Work 35
- Every Small Step Forward Counts 36
- You've Got This 36
  - Conclusion 37

Cope with the Stress of Dyslexia 38
- Don't Compare Yourself to Anyone Else 42
- Embrace a Positive Outlook 43
- Quiet Your Inner Critic 44
- Build Your Confidence 45
- Have Compassion for Yourself 46
- Lean into What Makes You Unique 47
- Strategies to Improve Your Mental Health 47
- Conclusion 55

Improve Your Literacy Skills 56
- Dyslexic Adults Can Have a Variety of Literacy Challenges 57
- It's Never Too Late to Improve Your Reading 60
- The Orton-Gillingham Approach 61
- What Is Phonological Awareness? 62
- Literacy Encompasses a Range of Skills 63
- Practice, Practice, Practice! 65

Strategies to Improve Your Literacy	65
Conclusion	74
Sharpen Your Auditory, Visual, and Spatial Skills	**75**
Auditory Perception and Discrimination Challenges	76
Visual Perception and Discrimination Challenges	78
Spatial Awareness	80
Remember, Everyone Is Different	81
Strategies to Improve Your Auditory, Visual, and Spatial Skills	82
Conclusion	89
Master Your Executive Functioning Skills	**90**
What Role Does Executive Functioning Play in the Body/Mind?	91
What Are the Executive Functioning Challenges for a Dyslexic Individual?	96
The Key Is to Know Yourself	99
Strategies to Improve Your Executive Functioning	100
Conclusion	110
Embrace Your Strengths	**111**
There Are Many Inherent Strengths That Come with Dyslexia	112
You Can Use These Skills to Your Advantage	117
Society Is Slowly Embracing Neurodiversity	117
Workplaces and Schools Are Becoming More Accommodating	117
Building Up Your Strengths Will Help Boost Your Confidence	119
Strategies to Build Your Strengths	119
Conclusion	129
Spelling	131
Formulating Words	132

Mild Social Anxiety	132
A Philanthropic Support Group	133
Build It and They Will Come	134
Planning an Event	134
Filling Out a Job Application	135
Improv	136
Accessing Your Intelligence	137

CHAPTER 1

Let's Talk about Dyslexia

What exactly is dyslexia? You may have heard that dyslexia means seeing letters move on the page or that it's exclusively a reading issue. The truth is dyslexia is more complex than that. While some characteristics are shared, dyslexia looks a little different in each of us who have it. In this chapter, we will attempt to define dyslexia and clear up some common misconceptions. You will be able to recognize the challenges of living with dyslexia, including some you may not have considered before. And with a clearer understanding of how dyslexia operates in your life, you'll be ready to move forward and make changes for the better.

TALIA

Talia was in her first year of law school when she reached out to me. The amount of reading required in her studies seemed beyond her capability. Talia had always been a slow reader and an abysmal speller. Throughout her school career, Talia had needed to work much harder than her peers. Until now, she had been able to handle the extra workload it took for her to be an A/B student. But this time she was at risk of failing her coursework.

    Although confident in her high verbal and analytical skills, in law school Talia struggled to organize the information she was expected to learn. Many of her tests used the format of short answer essays or multiple-choice questions. Talia found multiple-choice tests particularly difficult. She preferred the short answer tests, but even with those she was unable to express her thoughts in the allotted time. Talia felt her scores would better represent her knowledge if she were allowed more time to complete the tests.

Once she was diagnosed with dyslexia, Talia was granted extended time on tests. She was also provided a notetaker for her lecture courses. While an anonymous student jotted down key points during lectures, Talia was able to listen and make mental connections between the topics being presented. Talia also utilized digital textbooks, enabling her to hear complex words and sections read aloud. Hearing difficult words read correctly made it easier for Talia to recall terminology and case names. Talia passed her coursework and eventually her state's bar exam.

What Is Dyslexia?

Let's review some basic facts.

Dyslexia is defined as a language-related learning difference that is neurologically based and makes reading, writing, and spelling exceedingly tricky. This is reflected in the name of the condition: In Greek, dys means "difficulty," and lexia means "language." So the term dyslexia translates as a difficulty in processing language.

Although it varies in degrees of severity, dyslexia is common, more common than many people realize. It's generally reported that about 15 percent of the population has dyslexia, which adds up to over 30 million people in America.

The defining feature of dyslexia is the unexpected challenges in reading and spelling that it brings, challenges that seem to fly in the face of how smart we are. When not addressed, this gap between abilities and language skills can do significant damage to one's confidence and self-esteem.

What Dyslexia Isn't

Since there are many misconceptions about dyslexia, let's rule out some of them.

Dyslexia is not:

- Seeing letters backward or jumping all over a page of text

- Lacking instruction in phonics
- A medical condition

You should also know that dyslexia is not due to low intelligence or lack of motivation. Dyslexia is not exclusively a reading problem or unique to English language users.

And, as we've said, dyslexia is not rare. Fifteen to 20 percent of the general population are believed to have dyslexia. If you have dyslexia, you are not alone!

What Causes Dyslexia?

Dyslexic brains are wired differently.

Brain imaging techniques like magnetic resonance imagery (MRI) have revealed that reading involves multiple cognitive processes. Effective readers utilize three dominant areas of the brain during reading:

Broca's area, located in the brain's frontal lobe, is essential for speech production and articulation. This part of the brain connects sounds to letters.

The parietotemporal area is responsible for word analysis and for deciphering new words.

The occipitotemporal area of the brain activates to read words rapidly; this is where the brain retains mental images of word forms—that is, what a written word looks like.

Compared to the general population, people with dyslexia overuse their Broca's area when they read and don't engage the parietotemporal or the occipitotemporal areas. Their brains are not wired to read efficiently; they don't access the mental resources that non-dyslexic readers use.

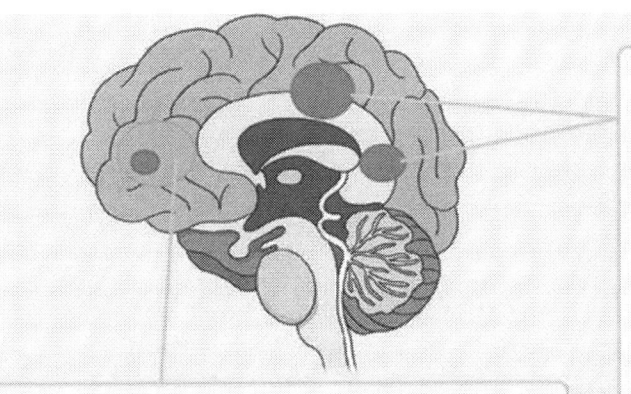

Broca's area: People with dyslexia primarily overuse this part of the brain (grey). They can recognize the sounds letters make—phonics.

However, people with dyslexia do not readily activate these areas of the brain to read, the parieto- and occipitotemporal areas. Pathways to these areas are underdeveloped in the dyslexic brain. (Efficient readers use the blue parts.)

Is There a Genetic Component?

Dyslexia runs in families, but the genetic link to dyslexia is complicated. No single gene can identify a risk for dyslexia. In fact, several genetic variants are linked to reading ability and literacy.

Having a family member with dyslexia increases your risk for dyslexia, but it's not the only factor. Research on identical twins revealed that 30 to 40 percent of the time, only one twin develops dyslexia. When a child is diagnosed with dyslexia, it is likely that one parent, sibling, or close relative has dyslexia too, though it may never have been identified. But having a family member with dyslexia does not mean you will develop dyslexia.

Famous Figures with Dyslexia

People with dyslexia are disproportionately found in careers requiring creative, out-of-the-box thinking. You might recognize some of these names:

CEOs and Entrepreneurs

Richard Branson, owner of Virgin airlines, credits dyslexia for his greatest strengths. Charles Schwab discovered he was dyslexic when his son was diagnosed; he reports having trouble with the alphabet even now.

Actors

Henry Winkler and Whoopi Goldberg struggled to read their scripts. Both report being able to memorize their lines. Cher speaks about her struggle with reading and numbers in her autobiography The First Time.

Athletes

Muhammad Ali, Tim Tebow, and Magic Johnson report never giving up despite dyslexia-related challenges. In fact, Johnson says his struggle spurred him on to do better. Michelle Carter, a three-time Olympian and 2016 Gold Medalist, reports never being shy about her dyslexia and ADHD.

Authors

F. Scott Fitzgerald and Agatha Christie both were avid readers but terrible spellers and likely had dyslexia. Max Brooks, author of The Zombie Survival Guide and World War Z, acknowledges that accepting his dyslexia has been important for his stories.

Nobel Prize Winners

Molecular biologist Carol Greider (2009), chemist John B. Goodenough (at age 97, 2019), and poet William B. Yeats (1923) have all recognized the struggles and the advantages that came with having dyslexia.

Why Is Dyslexia So Misunderstood?

Until recent decades, little was known about dyslexia. While psychiatrists and educators recognized that dyslexia involved the brain processing words differently, the general population only spotted the symptoms. In its early years, what we now call dyslexia was termed "word-blindness" by a German physician. As early as 1887, German physicians recognized that some people had trouble reading despite being bright, motivated, and educated.

Fast forward to the early 1980s in the United States. In those days, a reading disability was only recognized when a student was severely below grade level. Teaching methodology in reading ignored the possibility of diverse brain structures. Then the first clinical studies identified dyslexia in one out of five children. Many students with dyslexia had been compensating for their weaknesses with other intellectual strengths, such as visual-spatial skills, problem-solving aptitude, and creativity. They, and maybe you, secretly suffered and needed to work twice as hard as their peers to attain a passing grade.

By the mid-1990s, scientific data proved what early researchers had observed: Dyslexia is a neurological disability. Likewise, research studies confirmed that treatment of dyslexia through specialized instruction can impact how a brain processes language. As of March 2020, 46 states have passed legislation relating to dyslexia and education. Today, nonprofit organizations continue promoting dyslexia awareness.

The Key Features of Dyslexia

Dyslexia is a difficulty with decoding and spelling words. Decoding is the ability to use letter-sound relationships to understand a printed word. Likewise, a person with dyslexia will likely have challenges in speech and written communication. Many individuals with dyslexia can learn to read without any specific teaching methods to compensate for their dyslexia. Still, they will likely be unable to decode words they haven't seen before the way a non-dyslexic reader can.

Because reading takes so much brain energy, comprehending what one reads can become increasingly difficult as reading material becomes more challenging. We call this effect the third-grade wall, because in that grade words and sentences become longer and young readers can no longer use the word shapes and cues in the passage to comprehend text meaning. A student with dyslexia might appear to be reading. But if you listen closely, you'll notice they make minor errors when reading aloud. By adulthood, the effort it takes to read impacts reading comprehension.

Processing Difficulties Related to Dyslexia

Weak phonological processing is the hallmark of dyslexia. Phonological processing is how one detects and discriminates sounds in their language. It's an ability made up of three components, each of which is required for efficient reading skills:

Phonological awareness is being able to identify the most minor sounds that a word is composed of and understanding how those sounds interact to form words.

Phonological memory is the brain's ability to process and use information for reading and language. This working memory must combine sounds to form words, command words to produce sentences, and retain sentences to comprehend the whole meaning.

Finally, to be skillful readers, our brains must process information quickly through rapid naming. This requires the brain to rapidly take in visual data, retrieve meaning from stored knowledge, and attach a name to the image of a word on a page.

Dyslexia May Overlap with Other Learning Disorders

One of the complexities of managing dyslexia is that its symptoms commonly overlap with or mimic those of other conditions. Likewise, dyslexia symptoms can coexist alongside those of another disorder. Unfortunately, no blood test or MRI can pinpoint the exact learning disorder at play, so a diagnosis can be challenging if multiple disorders are present.

It is often tricky to distinguish one from another. For example, both dyslexia and attention deficit hyperactivity disorder (ADHD) can cause poor reading skills. Both can produce inaccurate, choppy oral reading. However, the dyslexic reader has difficulty with sounding out a word. In contrast, the ADHD reader may make mistakes due to poor impulse control or lack of focus. ADHD and dyslexia commonly coexist, and having both can exacerbate symptoms.

To be diagnosed with a learning or attention disorder, including dyslexia, one must have persistent symptoms over time and in different environments (i.e., not just at home or just at work or school). Also, distinctive signs of the disorder must have been identified in more than one developmental stage.

Let's review some of the disorders that can exist with dyslexia or be confused with it.

ADHD

ADHD (attention deficit hyperactivity disorder) is a neurological disorder that makes it difficult for someone to regulate their attention and maintain self-control. Some people with ADHD experience higher hyperactive and impulsive behavior, while others may only experience distractibility. And some people will have combined symptoms, both hyperactivity/impulsivity and distractibility. Indicators are judged on the severity with which they impact one's everyday life. To be diagnosed with ADHD in adulthood, symptoms must have been present in childhood.

Dysgraphia, Dyspraxia, Dyscalculia

Remember, dys refers to difficulty. Some learning disorders are named similarly to dyslexia:

- Dysgraphia is difficulty with writing.
- Dyspraxia is a physical difficulty affecting motor control.
- Dyscalculia is difficulty with math.

Like dyslexia, all these disorders are neurological and not related to intelligence. Each has multiple indications that can occur separately or alongside other disorders. For example, dysgraphia can be identified through poor handwriting, having difficulty putting words on paper, or inconsistent spelling, but it isn't due to a phonological deficit. Dyspraxia can manifest in adults as low muscle tone, poor posture, or fatigue. Dyscalculia stems from a conceptual weakness in problem-solving and calculating math.

How Do You Receive a Diagnosis?

No single test can diagnose a learning disability, including dyslexia. Typically, academic skills, visual-motor integration, and processing abilities are evaluated. The combined tests are analyzed to reveal struggles with word-level reading and spelling. In Sally Shaywitz's second edition of Overcoming Dyslexia, she emphasizes the importance of clinical judgment over arbitrary scores. There's no magic cut-off number that confirms dyslexia. A diagnosis should consider someone's academic, medical, and family history.

As we've said, the core of dyslexia is a phonological weakness (that is, difficulty processing the smallest element of sounds in spoken and written language). Children can be tested for this as young as four years old. Tests for adults might include checks of visual and auditory perception, discrimination, and memory. An intelligence test is not necessary; however, it can be a strong validation for bright individuals who have trouble reading.

If you suspect you have dyslexia but haven't been diagnosed, find a professional with experience assessing adults, an in-depth knowledge of dyslexia, and a broad understanding of language development and other disabilities. This professional does not need to administer the tests, but they must be qualified to interpret test results. A diagnostic report should include test results with interpretive summaries that are synthesized into an analytical conclusion, and it must be dated and signed.

The Importance of Early Intervention

Early intervention for dyslexia solves later academic problems and prevents people from developing low self-esteem and feelings of distress.

The risk of dyslexia can be observed in children at every developmental stage and addressed before a sense of failure develops. Screenings are recommended at the end of kindergarten and first grade for any child who shows indicators for dyslexia or has a family history. Unfortunately, most schools wait until third grade or later, by which point a student with dyslexia might already be failing school.

Catching dyslexia early makes a difference. Research shows overwhelmingly that students who receive intervention in first and second grades make remarkable reading gains. The US National Institutes of Health states that 95 percent of poor readers can be brought up to grade level via early intervention. That window of opportunity is kindergarten through first grade.

Best of all, the curriculum for students at risk for dyslexia will benefit all emerging readers.

A Late Diagnosis Means Additional Years of Stress and Frustration

When dyslexia goes unrecognized, the lateness of a diagnosis can pile unnecessary psychological problems on top of the struggle to live with dyslexia. For example, older students might avoid participating in class, lack motivation to study, or be resistant to interventions that might help them. Over time, negative emotions can impact all learning areas, making it harder for a student to overcome an achievement gap. Nevertheless, it is never too late to be helped. Once an individual receives the appropriate assistance, they can make substantial gains in two to three years.

Self-Assessment:
What Is Your Experience with Dyslexia as an Adult?

Everyone's experience with dyslexia is different, so let's pause to reflect on your own journey. Find a quiet place and time with your favorite hot drink. For this exercise and others in this book, you will need some form of journaling material to record your thoughts: pen and paper, a designated notebook, your laptop or digital device. Consider using a voice-to-text option if writing or typing is difficult for you. The purpose is to allow you time to reflect on why you are seeking information on dyslexia.

Record your answers to the following questions and prompts. When you're done, review what you recorded. Use the information to compose a narrative, a short story describing your dyslexia experience.

1. What is your history with dyslexia up to this point?
2. Examine your feelings about your education. Where were the pitfalls? What were the highlights?
3. Why are you pursuing an answer now?
4. Reflect on reading, writing, and processing challenges in your daily life.
5. List the reading and writing demands in your current job.
6. Do you recognize other learning disorders mentioned in this chapter comingled with your dyslexia?
7. Talk about the things you choose to do for pleasure.

When you're finished, title and save your narrative in a safe place to add to or revise later.

The Common Challenges of Dyslexia

The crux of dyslexia is a daily challenge in reading, writing, and spelling. However, these problems can show up in a multitude of daily trials. Due to insufficient phonological processing, someone with dyslexia can have trouble decoding an unfamiliar word they encounter in a book, article, or email. They tend to skip over unknown or long words when reading. Often their language difficulty can be observed in messy or unorganized handwriting.

Rote memorization is especially hard for dyslexics. Errors with directionality—mixing up right and left, misreading a map, flip-flopping terms like behind and in front—can be an issue at any age. A person with dyslexia may read a clock wrong or connect an appointment to the wrong day. Math might also be challenging, despite having higher-level thinking capabilities.

You may recognize some of the following daily challenges in yourself or your children. But knowing the core reason behind them can bring you a new understanding and a sense of relief.

Speech

Some of the earliest indications of dyslexia are found in speech. Stuttering and articulation issues can be early signs of dyslexia. Likewise, multisyllabic words can be mixed up; for example, helalopter or psghetti. Even adults might appear to have immature speech. A person with dyslexia may have trouble bringing up the words they intend to say on demand. Sometimes this is due to a lack of word-finding, the "It's on the tip of my tongue" feeling. Other times, someone with dyslexia may avoid using a particular word because they aren't confident in pronouncing it.

Reading and Writing

A person with dyslexia can read a word on one page but not recognize it on the next. In reading fluency, they may leave out functional words or replace unfamiliar words with synonyms or words that have similar patterns. Spelling is problematic; a student with dyslexia might study for hours and hours for school spelling tests but cannot retain the words a week later. While a person with dyslexia can hide or compensate for a reading problem, spelling difficulties tend to reveal themselves. Securing one's thoughts on paper may take an extraordinarily long time because of the need to avoid and correct spelling mistakes among other challenges.

Auditory, Visual, and Spatial Awareness

A weakness in auditory, visual, or spatial awareness identifies dyslexia across developmental stages. High intellect cannot typically mask someone's inadequacies in these areas. Spatial awareness problems can lead to mistakes relating to time or location: getting lost, showing up early or late to appointments, having trouble following GPS or mapping app instructions. Even telling time on an analog clock can be difficult. Someone with these issues might confuse left and right. When they're writing, placement of words on paper or inconsistent writing size can indicate cause for concern.

Executive Functioning

Executive functioning is the group of mental processes we use daily to learn, to work, and to manage our life. Due to insufficient language processing, someone with dyslexia may be challenged to sustain attention when reading or listening, which can lead to difficulties in executive functioning. Or they may have a tough time initiating or prioritizing tasks, knowing they'll have to work harder than most of their peers and will face extra challenges.

Stress, Low Self-Esteem, and Other Mental Health Issues

Unidentified dyslexia can cause psychological ramifications. Intrinsically, individuals with dyslexia believe that they can learn, yet their day-to-day difficulties lead to frustration and failure. With their self-esteem and confidence eroded, they may avoid opportunities in life. People with dyslexia are not typically depressed, but they do have a higher risk of sadness and anxiety. Instead of identifying the impacts of their disability, they tend to turn their anger on themselves.

Interesting Statistics on Adults with Dyslexia

Over 50 million people in the United States may have dyslexia. It is unknown how many adults have dyslexia, and sources vary widely in their estimation, with prevalence rates ranging from 5 to 20 percent. The International Dyslexia Association estimates that 15 to 20 percent of the population has some symptoms of dyslexia. The British Dyslexia Association states the number to be 1 in 10. No matter the exact percentage, experts agree that many adults with dyslexia go undiagnosed.

Dyslexia is the most common reason for a reading, writing, or spelling struggle. Research suggests that 70 to 80 percent of poor readers have dyslexia.

People with dyslexia can participate in higher education. In fact, according to the National Center for Learning Disabilities, 67 percent of high school graduates with a learning disability enroll in college, paralleling their non-dyslexic peers.

Dyslexia is well represented in the world of business and finance. According to a study by London's Cass Business School, 35 percent of entrepreneurs in the United States identify as dyslexic. According to John Chambers, former CEO of Cisco Systems, 25 percent of CEOs are dyslexic. Similarly, one comprehensive study showed 40 percent of the world's millionaires are dyslexic.

And though no statistics are available, many observers have noted that dyslexia is highly represented in creative fields such as architecture, engineering, and the arts.

The Inherent Strengths of People with Dyslexia

Leaders in the field recognize an aptitude for critical thinking, reasoning, and concept formation among people who have dyslexia. These kinds of inherent strengths are not necessary for a dyslexia diagnosis, but the notion that there is a bright side to dyslexia should be encouraging. Everyone has talent, and we shouldn't let dyslexia obscure that fact.

In their book The Dyslexic Advantage, Brock and Fernette Eide developed the acronym MIND to describe the gifts of dyslexia in terms of four categories:

Material reasoning, or creativity
Interconnected reasoning, or connectiveness
Narrative reasoning, or imagination
Dynamic reasoning, or intuition

While the academic challenges of dyslexia are real, the Eides have turned the conversation to the abilities or gifts of dyslexia, arguing that dyslexic strengths can be a trade-off for the challenges.

Creativity

There has been a longtime belief that people with dyslexia can easily imagine things in three dimensions, an upside to having strong spatial awareness. While there is some validity to this, not all dyslexics can instinctively visualize three-dimensional models. However, some with dyslexia do report being able to perform intricate designs in their head, despite routinely confusing two-dimensional letters and number shapes. This and other positive attributes of dyslexia are not always appreciated in younger years, which is one reason highly creative people with dyslexia generally blossom later in life.

Connectiveness

Many people with dyslexia report the ability to connect with people through relationships. They're described as empathetic, understanding diverse perspectives. They're good at connecting ideas, too. As scholars, people with dyslexia tend to delve into multiple disciplines. They are big picture thinkers, not studying anything in isolation but instead connecting bits of information to form big ideas. They miss the trees but see the forest. For example, Douglas Merrill, first CIO of Google and a person with dyslexia, has said, "I've always been interested in the overlap between psychology, sociology, and history."

Imagination

Surprisingly, despite their childhood struggles to learn to read and write, some of our greatest storytellers have dyslexia. The brain areas that recall personal events through episodic memory can be well developed, or gifted, in some of these writers and storytellers. They're skilled at remembering the past, understanding the present, and creating imaginary scenes. This kind of imagination is not limited to writers. Many actors, teachers, and politicians with dyslexia are applauded for their creative minds.

Intuition

The definition of intuition is the ability to understand something immediately, without the need for conscious reasoning. People in this category use the dyslexic strength of perceiving subtle patterns in complex systems in order to make predictions. As children, their apparent indifference to minute details may have seemed like wasting time and a disinterest in learning. In fact, they grow up to be our CEOs, entrepreneurs, and strategists—our problem solvers. Intuition has enabled many people with dyslexia to contribute considerably to society.

Dyslexia Affects Everyone Differently

Most people associate dyslexia with challenges that center on school or work. But dyslexia does not stay in the office or classroom. While following directions using Google Maps, someone with dyslexia might turn left instead of right. A busy mom might have difficulty planning the time between her appointments, resulting in being late for everything. When one dyslexic gives another dyslexic their email address, their emails will probably never reach each other. Spell check does not recognize the word you mean to type, so you have to look it up on Google. You can't even spell dyslexia. Hopefully, one can laugh at these dyslexic moments; nonetheless, they do complicate daily life.

Some scenarios are more significant and cause emotional scars. For example, a college student might be asked to read aloud and stammer, causing embarrassment and shame. Similarly, an administrative assistant may have difficulty organizing their thoughts when replying to an email, impeding progress in other areas of their workload. The result is stress and, ultimately, anxiety.

Let's Figure Out What Works for You

There is no single approach to overcoming dyslexia. But dyslexia cannot be ignored. One thing that all proficient individuals with dyslexia have in common is they have embraced their dyslexia. By doing so, they could find work-arounds, accept support, and push for accommodations to achieve their goals. Remember the stories of famous figures with dyslexia earlier in this chapter? There are many more encouraging stories of accomplished people speaking about the hard challenges and the benefits of having dyslexia in their lives. In the upcoming chapters, we'll share some as we figure out what works for you.

You Can Successfully Manage Your Dyslexia (But There Is No Cure)

Embracing your dyslexia means accepting that dyslexia is a lifelong condition. Although many learn to live, and thrive, with the symptoms, there is no cure. Accepting this, many people grow to appreciate their own characteristics that are associated with and connected to their dyslexia. The key to living with dyslexia is to lean on your strengths while sharpening your weaknesses. When a shortcoming cannot be refined, minimize it, but do not hide it. Embrace the picture of dyslexia in your life. Don't be afraid to say, "Oh, that's just my dyslexia."

There is no quick fix to managing dyslexia. Like our own brain, most of the plans we make for living with dyslexia will need to adapt to the changing demands of everything from a new job to a growing family. Dyslexia is not just a reading and writing problem. Symptoms can be wide-ranging; no one will display all signs at once. Most importantly: Bright, accomplished individuals can have dyslexia. A person with dyslexia might struggle in one career and excel in another. As the condition evolves over your lifetime, its symptoms will have a different impact at various stages of your life. Barriers can be overcome; putting a name to your struggle is the first step.

What Are Your Goals?

Let's continue the personal narrative you began earlier in this chapter. Now that you know more about the strengths and challenges commonly attributed to dyslexia, take some time to reflect on the impact dyslexia has had on your life, both the good and the bad. Then answer the questions listed below, using whatever journaling format you started in the previous exercise. This time, our purpose is to survey what's ahead and consider what you might achieve.

1. What challenges listed in this chapter did you most relate to?
2. Think of a dyslexic moment you have experienced; refer back to the list of challenges if needed. Try to pick an event you can laugh about. If you're comfortable, admit an event that caused embarrassment. Describe it in your journal.
3. Look back on the challenges you identified in the first reflection. What reading and writing skills do you expect to improve as you learn to manage your dyslexia, and why? What outcome do you hope to have?
4. What inherent strengths can you identify in yourself? Share an example that demonstrates one or more gifts in your life.
5. Consider interests that you've avoided in the past because of low confidence or self-esteem. Which ones would you most like to pursue?
6. What do you hope to achieve by reading this book? Pick three to five specific goals you wish to accomplish by the time you reach the last chapter.

This Book Will Show You How

If you display signs or symptoms of dyslexia, this book is for you. In the upcoming chapters, we'll identify dyslexia's hidden challenges, offer solutions, and steer you toward discovering your inherent strengths.

In chapter 2, we'll explore the unique difficulties of navigating dyslexia in adulthood. Then, chapters 3 to 6 will consider the routine aspects of managing those difficulties, empowering you with practical resources and strategies. In chapter 7, we'll celebrate the strengths that your dyslexia has granted you, and we'll finish in chapter 8 by observing some specific scenarios that depict how dyslexia manifests in the real world.

Throughout the book, you will be guided to reflect and discover. Never forget that whatever your academic challenges, you were born with an innate desire to learn and the tenacity to do so. I trust these pages will spark a desire for ongoing inquiry about your dyslexia, via this book and the other resources. By doing so, you'll take ownership of your dyslexia. And inspiring you to do that is my greatest aspiration.

Conclusion

Dyslexia is a common condition, but it's complex. Scientists have been studying what it is and how to treat it for centuries. Even so, over just the past two decades, we've come to know more about dyslexia than ever before. That's exciting! Many accomplished people have dyslexia and are outspoken about it.

Despite this broadening awareness, you may have felt misunderstood since childhood. School may not have felt safe to you, and adult struggles of everyday life can be extra tricky with dyslexia in the picture. It is vital to keep in mind that you are not alone.

In the next chapter, we will explore the dual nature of dyslexia: It brings us both strengths and weaknesses. As adults, we can choose to leverage our strengths to the fullest and not let our weaknesses hold us back. With that mindset, the possibilities become limitless.

CHAPTER 2

Navigate Dyslexia as an Adult

Now that you have a grounding in the facts about dyslexia, in this chapter we'll consider the different ways in which those truths can manifest in your life. We'll discuss ways that you can advocate for your needs in school, home, or work. And along with the challenges that adults with dyslexia might face, we'll examine the upsides and opportunities.

LISA

My client Lisa is not embarrassed to disclose her dyslexia to others socially, but at work she's had mixed experiences. Lisa has felt labeled and judged at times because of the everyday challenges caused by her dyslexia. Lisa puts her heart and soul into her job as a county sheriff. Still, at times she feels limited by aspects of dyslexia. "It's not all about effort," she told me.

As Lisa shared her story, she grew emotional. Preparing for her sergeant's exam, an extensive timed multiple-choice test, Lisa is required to memorize many unconnected details and codes. Lisa is exceptionally reliable at her job and acknowledges her gifts of multitasking, problem-solving, and shuffling tasks. I'll add creativity, caring, and compassion to that list. Lisa excels at visualizing possibilities from various perspectives. However, a multiple-choice test cannot assess these talents. She'd be better explaining multiple solutions to scenarios presented to her. But the testing system is not in her favor, and she's concerned she won't be recognized for her capabilities on the job.

To bolster her confidence, Lisa reminds herself that she's been able to find work-arounds to her daily tasks, with positive results. She's always placed herself in jobs that rely on her strengths and been able to

> rely on support from partners and technology. As Lisa considers her upcoming test, she realizes that it's just another hoop. She has jumped through others before, and she always lands on her feet.

How Does Dyslexia Show Up in Adulthood?

A person with dyslexia reads substantially slower than their peers. By adulthood, most people with dyslexia can recognize words. However, they're prone to mistakes in substitution, omission, or transposition of letters in their oral reading. They may interpret a word incorrectly without realizing it.

As Sally Shaywitz points out in Overcoming Dyslexia, the problem is with word retrieval, not thinking. In fact, comprehension is a strength for someone with dyslexia. People with dyslexia use cognitive abilities in reasoning, often have an excellent vocabulary, and can deploy logic to connect ideas. Many possess a high level of analytical skills and excel at outside-the-box thinking. Nonetheless, they may need to read something several times to retain the information. Many prefer listening to audiobooks.

A person with dyslexia may talk around a word, lacking the precision for correct pronunciation. They commonly use simple vocabulary or vague terms to avoid saying the wrong word. Their spoken vocabulary is disproportionally simplistic compared with what they comprehend.

Often adults with dyslexia find they can use better vocabulary in writing than in speech. But organizing their thoughts into cohesive communication can be challenging. Technology helps, but in some cases spellcheck is not enough to prevent or correct errors.

Common Signs and Struggles

By adulthood, daily challenges reflect the complex history of struggling to read and spell imposed by dyslexia. Adults may experience one or more of the challenges in the diagram here. Each person has their own list of challenges and abilities. But all adults with dyslexia will experience some of those struggles.

At times, a person with dyslexia may also have trouble telling their left from their right or difficulties navigating directions even when using a map.

Memory

Rote memory is nearly impossible for someone with dyslexia; they must associate new information with longstanding knowledge to retain random facts. For example, a date in history, like July 4, 1776, has no meaning on its own to someone with dyslexia. Nevertheless, some dyslexics are historians who can remember details about past experiences and events and connect them into a narrative or story.

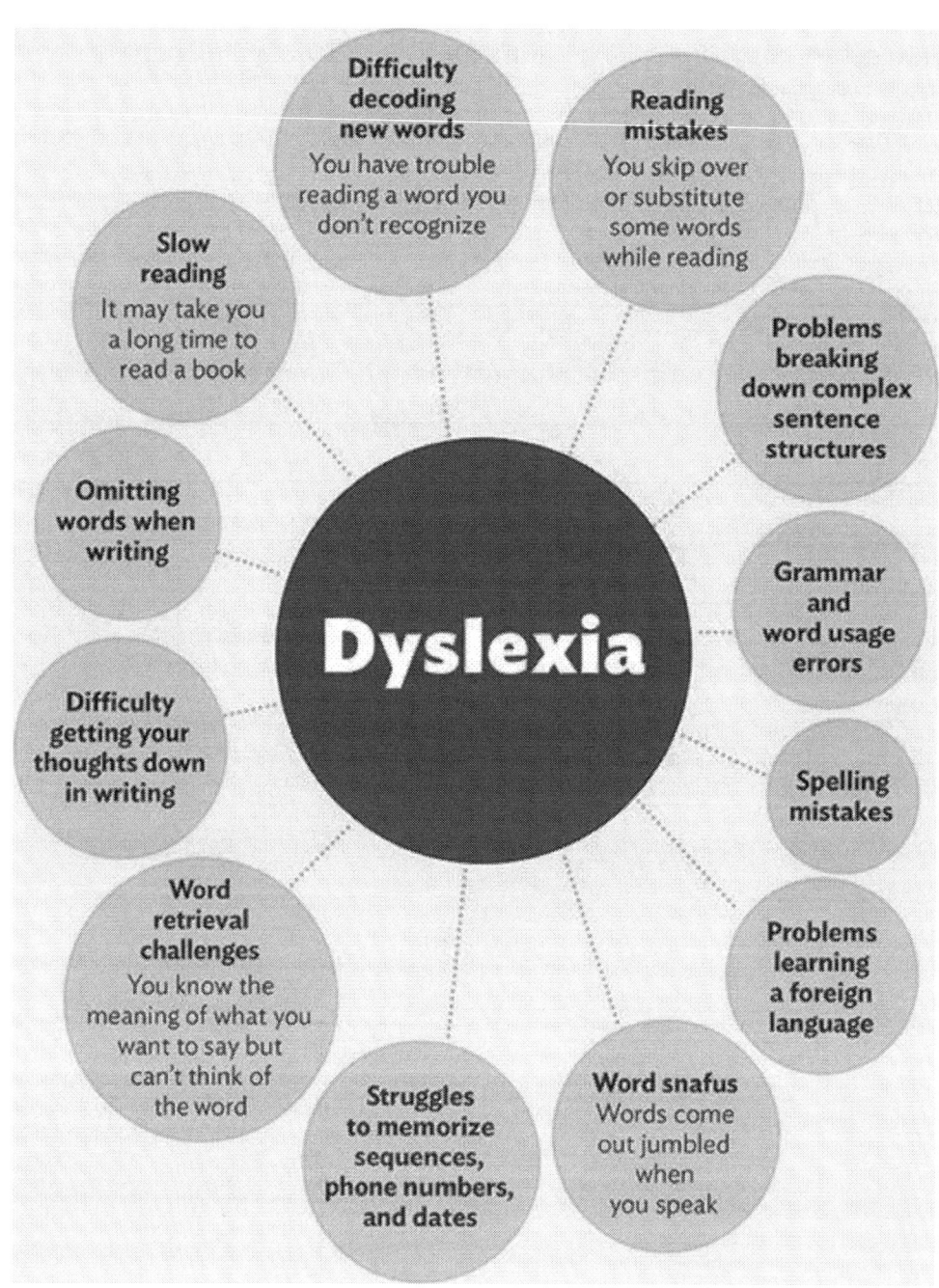

You May Have Been Struggling for Years without Knowing It

Dyslexia can be hidden, even from ourselves. The struggle might not be recognized until you reach a challenge you cannot compensate for, like your job suddenly requiring more reading and writing and less personal connection than before. Or you might observe a familiar battle in your child. Some people aren't aware of how much harder they've had to work compared with their peers. In my experience, when given an answer to a hidden struggle, adults are relieved to finally discover a reason and to put a name to it.

As one example, upon hearing his diagnosis of dyslexia, my client Anthony cried. Deep down, he had always suspected a problem. Anthony worked ridiculously hard to be successful, but a nagging inner voice questioned if he was as bright as his peers. Although he loved his job, he never felt safe. It turned out Anthony was, in fact, superior in intelligence to most of his colleagues. Finally, this adult had an answer for why he had to struggle so much with tasks that seemed easy for other people. You will hear more of Anthony's story in chapter 3.

Being an Adult Is Hard; Dyslexia Can Make Navigating Adulthood Harder

Adulthood comes with lots to juggle. Each stage of adult life brings challenges and blessings. It's important to remember that even adults without dyslexia find adulthood challenging at times. However, adults with dyslexia do carry an extra burden. Actress and singer Bella Thorne describes it this way: "Dyslexia makes things hard for me, but not impossible . . . I've learned to face problems, not run away from them."

If you've been living with dyslexia, emotional baggage that often accompanies years of overcompensation and expectations is bound to impact your self-confidence. By adulthood, you've needed to expend countless extra academic hours to do your best work. Feelings of shame and anxiety are familiar to adults with dyslexia and can contribute to low self-confidence and underachieving. We'll discuss the emotional impact of living with dyslexia in the next chapter. For now, take heart in knowing that although it may take you longer than other people to reach your goals, you've developed tremendous perseverance resulting from a lifetime of obstacles.

Work/Career

Adults with dyslexia have a lot to offer to the workforce. Contrasting with their school years, adults with dyslexia can design their own lives and pursue careers that honor their talents and personal qualities. However, dyslexia may still bring unexpected moments at work. You might feel shame or embarrassment, which can complicate work relationships. You might avoid certain tasks, which could make it harder to meet your responsibilities.

College

Your college years can be a great time to explore interests and develop your intellectual abilities. You'll find it easier to use technology and claim extended testing time to accommodate slow reading and abysmal spelling. However, college-level courses have more demands for note-taking and written expression. Organizing essays requires an extraordinary amount of work. And perfectionism can lead to performance anxiety and procrastination.

The Need for Extended Time on Tests

Current research has shed light on the need that students with dyslexia have for more time during testing. A recent study by dyslexia researcher Sally Shaywitz showed that adult college students used less efficient neural pathways when identifying words while reading. It takes an adult with dyslexia a long time to identify a word, but eventually most can correctly read a word that's in their vocabulary.

> While adult college students with dyslexia can read many words, they read them very slowly. In fact, they read more slowly than their sixth-grade counterparts, needing the extra time to use their higher cognitive skills and context clues for word identification. If given the extended time they need, these students can comprehend at the college level and perform at their intellect level.
>
> Here's the point: If you have dyslexia, you need more time to complete a test. Following a diagnosis, request extended time for board-certifying exams and for course exams and standardized tests in college and postgraduate school.

Family and Friends

People closest to you may notice your struggle, even if you haven't admitted it to them, and they may offer various unhelpful reactions with sound intentions. They might suggest that if you just try hard enough, you'll be able to read or spell as well as they do. They might get frustrated when you mispronounce a word. They may try to help you in public, drawing more attention to you and your snafu.

It's probably been hard for you to understand the impact that dyslexia has on your life; you may even be new to identifying it. So remember that it can be even harder for friends and family to get a handle on what you're going through. In some cases, shame due to unresolved feelings about your dyslexia may impede your ability to be vulnerable. This can make it challenging to form meaningful relationships. Outgoing personalities may find it more comfortable to focus on less intimate relationships, keeping to casual friendships until you feel your dyslexia is better managed.

Social Life

Adults with dyslexia might be shy, or they might be the life of the party. They might be self-centered or selfless. But however social you may be, a fear of being judged might block spontaneous expression in social settings. A game of charades could be a nightmare. A minor comment from someone after a flub might cause a downward spiral of humiliation.

Afraid to read even a birthday card or menu aloud in social groups, adults with dyslexia can overthink social situations, no matter how much they may want to participate. It's no wonder that adults with dyslexia commonly develop social anxiety.

Daily Responsibilities

Sometimes, you just have to laugh at the snafus dyslexia causes in daily life. For instance, I've shown up on the wrong day twice for the same dental appointment. Before everything was automated, I could not balance my checkbook because I easily transposed numbers or would round to the dollar, all this despite graduating with a finance degree. But in all seriousness, because daily reading and writing tasks take up so much time, between work and home life, people with dyslexia tend to have less free time available.

Young adults with dyslexia often take longer to find an interest to pursue, in some cases due to emotional scars. Childhood experiences may leave them with low self-esteem and low confidence. They may need extra years to achieve educational goals. Also, someone with dyslexia will typically look at all angles of a situation, so it can take them longer to commit to life milestones like choosing a career path. All of this can make it seem like a young adult who has dyslexia needs more time to grow up, is immature for their age, or is unable to take on responsibility.

Personal Goals and Dreams

Because of a lack of confidence, an adult with dyslexia might choose a less desirable career or field of study. Their personal goals might appear out of reach because of low academic and processing skills. If you feel that poor academic performance is holding you back, consider that Einstein hated school. He was told he would never amount to anything. Thomas Jefferson struggled to read and write as a student. A young aspiring Walt Disney was told he was not creative enough. What would our world be without their contributions? Doubtless, many people with dyslexia were not as successful at proving naysayers wrong. But armed with an acceptance of your condition and appreciation for its gifts, you can tilt the odds in your favor.

> ## Open Up to Someone If You Feel Comfortable
>
> It can be hard to admit you need assistance. But obtaining help can be empowering and provide you with confidence. A tutor can help you develop your skills in reading and spelling. An educational therapist can help you build academic skills while addressing other issues. Talk therapy might offer a safe place for you to manage your internal struggles. Therapists trained in cognitive behavioral therapy (CBT) might also be able to coach you in improving executive functioning skills.
>
>   To determine what sort of help to request, start by determining your primary concern—for example, improving your writing skills. Then, identify your secondary challenge; maybe you'd like to develop stronger organizational skills. With those goals in mind, search for a professional who's trained and knowledgeable in your top-priority problem and who possesses knowledge of your secondary concern. In this case you might look for a writing tutor who also helps people set up their home office or writing space. Note that medical insurance does not generally cover academic skills but will cover psychotherapy. Check with your insurance plan for details on what they'll cover.
>
>   When inquiring about treatment, find out the therapist's background and style. The therapist should understand emotional issues, preferably those related to dyslexia. They must be aware of dyslexia and its potential impact. Ask about this when evaluating potential therapists, and don't be afraid to discuss a treatment plan. Studies show that in many cases, a person with dyslexia does not need to dwell on the problem; they need a plan that moves them forward.

Everyone Has Their Challenges and Their Gifts

In their book The Dyslexic Advantage, Brock and Fernette Eide refer to the flipside, or trade-offs, to each aspect of dyslexia. I call this the dual nature of dyslexia: Each talent has an opposing weakness. For example, understanding and viewing spatial relationships can be a gift of dyslexia. However, two-dimensional processing—like interpreting letters printed on a page—can be challenging.

Similarly, we've noted that people with dyslexia tend to be global thinkers. They innately grasp unexpected relationships and patterns. But this can mean having a tough time with multiple-choice questions on tests, because the broad thinker can always find some vague merit in each possible choice. Global thinkers can substitute one same-meaning word for another when reading without skipping a beat. But to a listener or teacher this comes across as a failure to read.

An "ah-ha" or eureka moment offers some of our best thoughts, and it tends to come when we let our conscious minds wander and allow concepts to percolate beneath our awareness. The person with dyslexia who's deep in subconscious thought may appear to be distracted or goofing off. In fact, this is when a mind loses focus and begins to wander, making room for big, insightful ideas.

Get Clear on What You Need to Succeed

The principal accommodation that helps a person with dyslexia is more time: to read, to write, to think. With dyslexia, you merely take longer to learn, process, and organize your thoughts. This is an especially essential concern for official tests of knowledge, such as college course exams and state licensing tests. On the job, you will need to be more efficient and organized than your peers.

To set yourself up to succeed, ask yourself, "What are my strengths and passions?" The same gift can be helpful in some situations and detrimental in others. First, identify what you are skillful at; for instance, maybe you excel at generating creative concepts in brainstorming sessions. Next consider how the talent might cause a misunderstanding or a problem: If there's an email thread asking for specific solutions to a granular problem, you might find it hard to narrow your thinking—and composing your reply might take most of the afternoon.

What's important is that you're not shy about seeking support for weaknesses that accompany your talents. In this example, maybe you share your thoughts with a colleague, face to face, for feedback before sending your reply. Or ask them to read a draft of your email.

How to Prioritize What You Need to Succeed

For this exercise, you will be adding to the journal narratives you created in chapter 1. Remember, try to use a voice-to-text option if writing by hand or keyboard is difficult for you.

Because you need ample time for language and processing tasks, you need to become a capable organizer of your time. Start by asking yourself: What's working, what needs to change, and what is distracting me? Use the prompts below to help you identify your needs, then make necessary changes to accommodate your priorities.

1. Consider your work or school environment. Which elements are working to enable you to meet your responsibilities? Which are not? Take your time and consider everything, big and small, from your daily schedule to the devices and software you use, to the objects you keep on your desk or in your bag.

2. Create a picture, or find one on the internet, that resembles each of your gifts. For example, a picture of a light bulb might represent your ability to come up with surprising ideas. Cut out the images and paste them to your journal. For inspiration, you might make copies and stick them to your bathroom mirror, fridge, workspace, or some other spot that you will naturally eyeball every day.

3. Brainstorm three or four challenges mentioned in this or previous chapters that impact your work and daily life. Reflect on the effect each has on your job, learning, or personal life.

Record your thoughts and save the document for later, as we explore strategies in future chapters.

Remember, You Are Your Best Advocate

Under the Americans with Disabilities Act (ADA), employers must be informed that an individual has a condition and may need accommodations to perform essential functions in their job. The law does not require individuals to disclose their disability; however, according to the ADA, "Employers are not required to accommodate an undisclosed disability."

Is it better to claim a not-apparent disability in the workplace or keep it private? There are arguments for both options. Some people feel they can avoid being labeled or that strong motivation can work around a weakness without a need to bring disability into the conversation. For example, one might communicate their dyslexia needs casually to an understanding boss by saying, "I learn better with visual aids." You might delegate certain tasks or ask colleagues for help. However, not disclosing your disability is risky. There might be a change in management, support, or expectations that prevent your work-around solutions.

Many employers are understanding and aspire to help employees who have dyslexia. Will your manager or HR department recognize that you have a lot to offer in your job? You be the judge. But be willing to point out that for your employer to benefit from your strengths, you will need dependable support.

The Americans with Disabilities Act and Reasonable Accommodations

Adults typically seek a dyslexia diagnosis for one of three reasons:

- To benefit from reasonable accommodations in their workplace or school under the Americans with Disabilities Act (ADA)

- To receive extended time for standardized tests
- To satisfy a personal need to know

According to the Americans with Disabilities Act of 1990, the severity of the symptoms and how they limit your work or school performance determine the necessary accommodations. You must initiate the conversation by telling your representative about your condition, what reasonable accommodations you are asking for, and why they will help.

So what does "reasonable accommodations" mean? According to the ADA National Network, it is "any change to the application or hiring process, to the job, to the way the job is done, or the work environment that allows a person with a disability who is qualified for the job to perform the essential functions of that job and enjoy equal employment opportunities."

If you are requesting reasonable accommodations under the ADA, contact your human resources department, student services for disabilities office, or the relevant testing agency and ask what documentation they require to recognize your disability. The Dyslexia Screening Test App, available from NeuroLearning.com, is a reputable online screening tool that provides a score indicating an overall risk of dyslexia-related challenges. Individuals receiving a positive result may request a Proof of Disability certification.

Communicate Your Needs

When asked about their dyslexia, many people find themselves without the words to explain. I suggest you develop a short personal statement describing how dyslexia appears in your life. Practice so you can repeat it easily when needed. Sandwich your struggles between the facts and your strengths. For example, you might start with a textbook definition, describe what you find challenging, and end with your talents.

Here's a template you can use, if needed:

"Dyslexia is a language-based learning difference that is neurological, and makes _____, _____, and_____ difficult for me. But like many people with dyslexia, I'm good at _____, _____, and ___ _."

Owning your dyslexia will aid you in communicating your needs, in your personal life and at work, with confidence.

When asking for accommodations, start by expressing what you appreciate about your job. Recognize what you have to offer: innovative ideas, problem-solving skills, strong relations with clients or vendors, whatever's relevant. Then, as a team player, address areas of concern and offer solutions.

Be mindful of your employer's perspective; they might wish to help but must consider costs. Offer economical solutions that improve your team's overall productivity. For example, you might discuss shifting job responsibilities so you and a coworker each primarily utilize your different strengths.

Surround Yourself with a Supportive Team

Consider a soccer team. Each player brings their own talents to the field. The goalie's job is quite different from that of the attacking midfielder. Similarly, you need to perceive yourself as bringing a specific value to the team. While you offer problem-solving, creativity, and innovative ideas, others might easily retain rote facts or be able to troubleshoot minute details. A supportive team member might be someone who can edit your writing or prescreen your inbox so you can focus on reading the information you need.

And in your personal life, consider the people closest to you. How can your talents support their endeavors? At the same time, be upfront with them about how they can care for yours. You've heard that opposites attract; is there someone in your life you could swap tasks with to better utilize your different abilities? It can also be nice to have some overlap in strengths. For example, my husband and I are both goal persistent. We can practice grace in supporting each other to reach our personal goals.

Don't overthink your relationships—picking friends to fill in the gaps in your own capabilities won't work. But do surround yourself with people who believe in you and whom you can believe in.

Make an Action Plan

How do we plan for a change, whether we want to stay in our current environment or explore something new? Day-by-day or long-term growth requires a map to succeed. The first step is to identify your goal or desired outcome. This may require some initial research; for example, if you're considering a career shift, you might talk to someone who's working in that field.

Next, ask yourself:

- What tangible actions or materials do I need to achieve my goal?
- What are my strengths?
- In what ways will I need support in pursuing this goal, and where will I search for help?
- How long do I expect my plan to take?

Finally, set milestones and visualize your success. Along the way, monitor, evaluate, and update the plan as needed. Do not be afraid to ask for assistance or consider accommodations. You may not be a great reader, but you bring other talents to the table. Lean on those talents as your strengths.

A Quick Breathing Exercise for Difficult Days

Breathing exercises can bring the brain and the body into a calm state. There are distinctive types of breathing exercises. Diaphragmatic breathing, described here, can be performed easily and discreetly. And over time, being able to manage stress offers expanded health benefits. Try this exercise:

1. Sit or lie in a comfortable position.
2. Relax your shoulders.
3. Breathe in through your nose, feeling your belly expand.
4. Purse your lips, the same as if you were blowing through a straw, and gently exhale.

Repeat this sequence until you feel your desired calmness.

You Will Always Be Dealing with Dyslexia

It's an unavoidable truth: Dyslexia is a lifelong condition. There is no cure. But there is good news. You have a lifetime to grow into your dyslexia.

Research has vastly expanded our understanding of dyslexia over the last two decades. These days, dyslexia is more understood and accepted by society. And more people, young and old, are identifying their differences. Whatever difficulties your dyslexia has brought you in life, now is your own opportunity to understand the challenges and welcome the prospects that having dyslexia creates.

As an adult, you've already been through what are typically the roughest times for someone with dyslexia—your school years. By picking up this book, you've set out on a path toward learning more about yourself and your unique way of processing the world around you. Similar to any challenge, managing dyslexia takes perseverance and dedication. By shifting your focus from what you can't do to what you can accomplish, you will flourish.

It Takes Dedication and Hard Work

With dyslexia comes gifts, including the trait of perseverance. By working harder than most of your peers, you've developed habits and discipline you may not yet recognize. While it is true that dyslexia cannot be cured, it needn't hold you back. You can develop abilities and reach your goals through hard work and determination.

Maybe you feel regret that you couldn't perform well in school. Benjamin Bloom, an educational psychologist, studied outstanding achievers. He found that most were not remarkable as children. Their talents were developed through training. An example is Thomas Edison, who biographers describe as an average child. Underdogs have been known to accomplish remarkable feats. Individual athletes, recognized as underdogs, are motivated to win even though they are not the expected victors. Bloom held a strong belief that everyone can learn if provided with the right conditions to learn.

What set Edison and many others apart was their intense drive to learn. Many people with dyslexia possess ferocious determination. To the adage "You can accomplish anything you set your mind to," I like to add: "It just might take you longer to accomplish it. But you will."

Every Small Step Forward Counts

The process of managing your dyslexia can be a long road. But it's a journey worth taking. I can personally attest to that in my own life, and I've heard many encouraging stories from others. Sometimes you may feel like you're not making progress. But you cannot know where a small step will eventually take you. And keep in mind what a wise person once told me: "You can't stay where you are. You are either moving forward or backward." The direction is up to you.

You've Got This

There is no better time to have dyslexia than right now. Technology is evolving exponentially to meet the needs of a more efficient and asynchronous world. Employers are acknowledging the gifts of dyslexia and the contribution people with dyslexia can make. I dare say, it is even trendy to identify and share dyslexic moments.

Whatever your situation is, if having dyslexia has taught you anything, it's taught you determination. You can do anything you set your mind to. So be creative in your imagination. Take the opportunities that are presented to you, no matter how small or how big. And be patient. Rome was not built in a day, but I'd argue that big picture thinkers played a role in building that eternal city.

Conclusion

In this chapter, we learned that even in childhood, the dual nature of dyslexia affects us with strengths and weaknesses. Yet outside the confines of school, one's talents are better recognized. Although there are noticeable similarities, each person with dyslexia exhibits their uniqueness. Given the opportunity, any adult with dyslexia can achieve their dreams.

In the next chapter, we will discuss the emotional aspects of dyslexia. Underpinnings of shame, low self-esteem, and anxiety are commonly attributed to lifelong struggles of dyslexia. However, it's not all negative. The effects of dyslexia can also prompt a strong sense of empathy and compassion for others. Embracing your dyslexia by tackling the emotional side is unquestionably the best tool in your toolbox for building your best self.

CHAPTER 3

Cope with the Stress of Dyslexia

In this chapter, we'll tackle the emotional side of dyslexia. There's no denying the impact that feelings of frustration, inferiority, and shame can leave on our sense of well-being. Nevertheless, in my work I've witnessed again and again the value of embracing dyslexia and leaning into one's attributes. I've watched countless people of all ages shift the effects of dyslexia in their favor.

ANTHONY

In his early 50s, Anthony was a math professor at a local university, popular because he related so well to his students. But he had a secret. Anthony had always struggled to read and to express himself verbally. He could successfully read or talk about anything math-related, since he'd memorized the words and vocabulary. However, outside the context of mathematics, Anthony struggled to retrieve the correct words and feared making a mistake whenever he had to speak.

After years of a personal struggle with anxiety, Anthony sought the help of a psychologist and was diagnosed with dyslexia. Surprised and relieved to discover a tangible reason for his shame and anxiety, he dove into finding out more about it. Anthony sought coaching to help him identify and embrace his communication style and social anxiety. He learned that he had the words he wanted to say but needed the confidence to retrieve them.

As Anthony embraced his dyslexia, he became an advocate for students in his classes who displayed unexpected struggles with language. Anthony also joined an adult Toastmasters group to confront his public speaking barrier, which broadened his word retrieval skills and confidence in speaking on various topics.

> Anthony had found his social voice. He even got engaged to be married. Anthony describes it this way: "I now understand my struggles and have a name for them: dyslexia. I am no longer afraid of being discovered."

There Is Also a Mental Health Component to Dyslexia

Mental health is a state of well-being that allows us the coping skills we need to traverse our daily life challenges. Feelings of failure from early elementary school can be a long-term impediment to good mental health. Imagine a happy, well-adjusted, verbal child who goes to school but, despite a strong desire to learn, cannot fulfill their parents' and teachers' expectations to read. By fourth grade, children who experience this conclude that the problem must be them—that they are stupid. This secret shame often continues into adulthood.

Secondary emotional overlays to dyslexia are not always significant mental health issues like depression or an anxiety disorder. But the emotional consequences can still be debilitating, especially when dyslexia is diagnosed late in life, or never at all. When symptoms don't pose an immediate threat, it can be easy to de-prioritize mental health issues. You may need to give yourself permission to work on your mental well-being.

Low Self-Esteem

Self-esteem is how we feel about ourselves. It's not surprising that children and adults with dyslexia are prone to lower self-esteem when compared with their typical-reading peers. Until they reach age 18, much of their waking hours are spent in a school environment that relies on reading, which most likely produced negative experiences. That leads to negative self-talk, anxiety, and lack of confidence. The resulting low self-esteem from all those years of feeling like a failure is challenging to heal.

Low Self-Worth

Self-worth is the value we place on ourselves in our world. Healthy self-worth has positive effects on self-esteem and vice-versa. Those who are resilient have high self-worth despite any negative external messages they're given. They feel the pain of failure but still know they are valuable. Keeping your focus on strengthening your talents can promote healthy self-worth that will carry you though feelings of failure and shame.

Stress and Anxiety

Researcher Sally Shaywitz tells us, "Virtually everyone who is diagnosed as dyslexic, whether it is a Yale student, an Uber driver . . . or a retired senior citizen, comes with a full load of anxiety." When the underpinnings of stress are not addressed, it can cause anxiety. For someone with dyslexia, addressing stress means accepting their condition and taking steps to handle the consequences. For example, test anxiety can be addressed with academic intervention and accommodations. Most people report less general stress once they identify the challenges that stem from dyslexia and take action to manage them.

Quick Tools for Stressful Situations

When day-to-day circumstances overwhelm you, you can take steps to offset the negative feelings. Below are six suggestions to calm and refocus.

Find your safe place. Imagine being somewhere you enjoy, maybe a beach, the mountains, or reading a book in your favorite chair. Try to evoke your safe place with all your senses. Can you hear the waves crashing or feel your comfy blanket?

> Take a break. Temporarily remove yourself from a stressful situation and re-center your confidence. Take the time to pour a cup of tea or coffee, go for a short walk, or just catch your breath in a calm place.
>
> Be kind. Treat yourself with kindness when you're having a tough moment. Say something nice to yourself, something you'd say to encourage a friend: "You got this!" Decide on a treat to enjoy once you navigate your moment of stress.
>
> Give yourself a hug. Wrap your arms across your chest, touching the opposite shoulders; lean back against a chair and apply gentle pressure with your hug. Soak in the warm sensation.
>
> Just breathe. Breathing helps you relax and regroup. Take a deep breath and evaluate the situation. Use the <u>conscious breathing exercise</u> in chapter 2 to bring your body to a relaxed state.
>
> Accept your guest. Welcome your troubling emotions and doubts into your mind as unwelcome visitors. Research shows this lessens their impact. Unwelcomed visitors are temporary. We tolerate them, then they leave, and so will unwanted emotions. Tomorrow will be better.

Shame

Shame is powerful but can be defeated. When I think of shame, I think of dyslexia advocate Ben Foss, who advises, "Choose hope, not shame." Foss went from special education to completing law and business degrees from Stanford, with his mother as his scribe. Foss describes shame as "a feeling that you're unworthy because of something you are. It's different from guilt, which is feeling bad about something you did, like stealing or cheating." In those moments when one feels humiliated or unable to fit social norms or expectations, shame is born. Shame is self-imposed, typically due to fear of not being good enough. However, shame can be defeated by reframing your beliefs; we'll describe this strategy at the end of this chapter.

Feeling Misunderstood

People with dyslexia often feel misunderstood and underestimated, especially during their years in school. You might have been working twice as hard as your peers, yet your parents and teachers thought you were being lazy. More advanced classes, in which your talents could have shined, were not offered to you. Not being recognized for our abilities and efforts can be incredibly painful and confusing. As Einstein said, "If you judge a fish by its ability to climb a tree, it will live its whole life believing it is stupid." All too often, people with dyslexia are made to feel like that fish.

Frustration

The adult with dyslexia has lived a lifetime of frustration: the frustration of being misunderstood, of lost opportunities. Jaxon, a former client of mine, described his frustration in his career as a firefighter, saying: "I am the quickest at responding to emergencies. I always know just what to do and keep my head in the game, but I cannot pass the EMT II test, so I will never make rank." I'm happy to say that Jaxon was wrong about that. After we diagnosed his dyslexia, he was allowed extended time to take his test and a tutor to help him prepare. He is now an EMT II.

Don't Compare Yourself to Anyone Else

It's tempting to compare ourselves to others. But when you do that, you take your eyes off your goal. You might be envious of others' attributes or accomplishments, especially if they appear to be earned with much less effort than your own. However, often we measure our everyday accomplishments against others' highlights, causing a sense of inferiority. This is called upward comparison. Ironically, upward comparison brings about a downward spiral. Social media has expanded our opportunities to obsess over others' biggest, most significant moments. Of course, people rarely post their down moments, which creates a skewed view of what's normal.

So, what are we to do? The key is to embrace your dyslexia. Be content with who you are and with your progress. And allow yourself to feel proud. You deserve it! Focus on your strengths; be thankful and celebrate others and their accomplishments without envy. If you use social media, join a group that focuses on people with dyslexia. Have a policy of only comparing yourself to you.

Embrace a Positive Outlook

There are two significant types of mindsets, according to Stanford psychologist Carol Dweck: growth and fixed. With a fixed mindset, you believe you were born with predetermined abilities and attributes. If you have a growth mindset, you believe that talents can be developed and changed over time through effort.

Someone with a growth mindset accepts new challenges and explores opportunities to grow. No one loves criticism, but a person with a fixed mindset takes criticism personally. Whereas someone in touch with their growth mindset takes criticism as an opportunity to do better. They understand that the criticism is directed at their work, not intended to attack them personally. Most of us shift between fixed and growth mindsets to some extent. But a growth mindset is an asset that helps us learn from our errors and gain new skills. In fact, employers often use questions in the interviewing process to determine whether a candidate views mistakes with opportunism or failure.

It's not uncommon for a feeling of inadequacy to overwhelm us as we take on new challenges. Many successful people with dyslexia share stories of visualizing success as a way of focusing on the positive. In other words, they imagine what their accomplishments will look like. Unfortunately, the inner voices that remind us of our shortcomings can be hard to refute. However, when we're considering new opportunities, a growth mindset embraces our positive attributes and encourages us to envision future accomplishments.

Own Dyslexia, Don't Let It Own You

Not owning your dyslexia makes it harder to manage your life, leaving you vulnerable and on edge. For most of us, coming to terms with the harmful effects of dyslexia in our lives will be our chief hurdle. Frustrated feelings from years or decades of prolonged failure has resulted in shame, anxiety, and low self-esteem. Without reason as to why we struggle, we blame ourselves instead of blaming the environment. Even in adulthood, we may still call ourselves dumb or stupid under our breath. You may feel stuck, convinced that this is as good as your life will get.

Not true! Success is possible.

Such intense negative feelings result from a lack of understanding. But knowledge brings relief. When you recognize and label the cause of your problems, instead of blaming yourself, you can move forward.

You must take ownership of—embrace—dyslexia in your life. This can feel overwhelming at first, especially when you're just beginning to recognize the difficulties brought about by dyslexia. Start by merely being open to the possibilities.

Here's the good news: Your past does not need to dictate your future. By owning your dyslexia, you put yourself in control.

Quiet Your Inner Critic

We all need to be honest with ourselves about our errors and shortcomings. Self-analysis can be a healthy tool for one's overall mental health. But being overly and unreasonably critical of oneself can be destructive to our self-worth. As adults with dyslexia, we are often our own worst critics, driving ourselves back to old feelings of shame and fear of being found out as an imposter. I cannot tell you how often I contemplate my day and cringe at an embarrassing moment. But I've learned to keep my inner critic from taking over. I once misused a word in an email—I typed condom for condemn. While this was an embarrassment for a time, I can laugh at my blooper now.

Keep your inner critic in its place by challenging your negative thoughts. Ask yourself: Why am I being self-critical? What triggered the criticism? Reframe your perspective on the situation. Try to identify the worry or concern that's driving this negativity, and make a plan to handle it. Or, if nothing can be done, set your worry aside. Distract yourself with music, self-care, or a creative outlet that will soothe you. A calm brain can better process events and draw healthier conclusions.

Build Your Confidence

Everyone doubts their abilities from time to time. Low self-confidence is not isolated to someone with dyslexia. But someone with dyslexia almost certainly struggles with confidence, especially when facing a new challenge.

However, I would argue that someone with dyslexia will always produce quality work, given time and support. The formula for building self-confidence is to recognize your potential, measure your progress, and believe in your future self. What is that one thing that makes you unique? Focus on what you're talented at, and build on that.

A Confidence-Building Exercise

In this exercise, you will focus on your strengths. Access your journal (from chapters 1 and 2), and title this entry "Bettering My Self-Esteem." If you wish, after answering the reflection prompts, challenge yourself to complete one or two practical applications listed below.

Note: This is the last journal exercise in this book. But I encourage you to continue adding your thoughts when you feel inspired and to review what you've recorded from time to time.

1. List your accomplishments. If you're not used to giving yourself credit, this may take some brainstorming. These do not need to be big moments; give each achievement that's important to you equal weight.

   Practical application: Create or update your resume or CV.

2. Embrace dyslexia in writing. Jot down your thoughts, or use speech-to-text, regarding the positive effects of dyslexia in your life.

   Practical application: Express your feelings about dyslexia to a safe mentor or friend, or develop your personal statement about dyslexia as discussed in chapter 2.

3. Scrutinize your work or school circumstances. Write or voice-to-text your thoughts on how you can make your school or workplace feel like a safe, productive place to you.

   Practical application: Take steps to create a supportive environment where you can be productive and confident.

Dyslexia can be a heavy, ongoing burden. Seek professional counseling if feelings of low self-worth, shame, or other mental wellness issues are overwhelming. It's okay to request help when you feel low or confused.

Have Compassion for Yourself

Because we've had to face challenges, many of us with dyslexia develop a strong sense of empathy and compassion for others. But that doesn't always include compassion for ourselves.

Research shows that the empathy we offer ourselves is strongly related to our well-being. Psychologist Kristin Neff has devoted her career to studying compassion. She reports that when we are self-critical, our body releases cortisol, a hormone that has unhealthy effects on our physical and mental well-being over time. When we reiterate our failures and disappointments, we stagnate in our pain and undermine our motivation. On the contrary, when we begin to feel safe or cared for, our body reduces cortisol and discharges feel-good hormones. When we think agreeably about ourselves, we are at our optimal to do our best.

One way we generate self-compassion is by examining the dialogue we have with ourselves. When you're being self-critical, ask yourself, Is that what I'd say to a loved one? Or even an enemy? Dr. Neff suggests treating yourself as you would a beloved friend. Employ self-kindness. Normalize your imperfections: You are not alone in making mistakes; you belong to a community of others who struggle with dyslexia. Believe in yourself. You are not lazy or selfish.

Lean into What Makes You Unique

You are unique! No one is identical to you. Consider the pieces of a jigsaw puzzle. No matter how many pieces there are, no two bear the same image. The diverse individual details all contribute to the whole. You are a piece of the puzzle of the community you live in, bringing one-of-a-kind value to your relationships and work. For example, your ability to consider multiple perspectives allows for empathy and compassion for others. Your problem-solving skills might identify an answer to a complex question; you might imagine the big picture while working alongside others who better identify the details.

Hopefully, you've begun to catalog your unique set of characteristics in these first few chapters of this book. One useful avenue for discovering your unique traits is through personality or strength testing. There are some online options for these included in the Resources list at the end of this book. If you are considering a career change, you might work with a trained psychologist or career coach who can administer such tests and interpret your profile.

Strategies to Improve Your Mental Health

We'll end this and the following chapters with strategies related to each chapter's topic. These suggestions are not meant to overwhelm you but to offer options to explore. The following suggested strategies focus on calming your brain and cultivating mindfulness.

#1. Art or Photo Journaling

BEST FOR: Boosting mood while reflecting and creating

People with dyslexia often cringe when they hear the word journaling, which may bring uncomfortable memories of searching your brain for words, many of which you couldn't spell.

Let's reframe journaling to leave reading and writing out of the process. Words are not necessary to express your thoughts and understand your emotions. Consider art or photo journaling as an alternative.

Research has shown that keeping a journal lowers blood pressure and increases immune system functioning. Journaling can also boost mood, improve cognitive processing, and expand your self-awareness.

Here are some steps to get you started:

1. Decide on your medium: drawing, photography, digital images, etc.
2. Collect whatever supplies you need.
3. Dedicate a convenient journaling space. Keep materials where you can easily access them. Remember, daily journaling offers the most benefits.
4. Decide on a theme. Give your journal a title, or put a description on the first page. You might want a broad topic, like your journey with dyslexia, or something more specific, like representing something you saw during the course of each day.
5. Consider ways to fuse different media or elements: illustrations with words cut out from magazines; drawings with photographs; collages of found objects, like stickers or comic strips or menus. There are no rules!

Most of all, let your creativity loose and have fun. Journaling offers a way to reflect the complexity of what is in your head. It's unique to you.

#2. Relaxing with Color

BEST FOR: Reducing stress

Adult coloring books have become exceedingly popular. Overwhelmingly, my adult clients recommend coloring books for cultivating mindfulness (more about that in strategy #10). Working with color can be soothing and calms the brain. Some ancient cultures have attributed healing benefits to certain colors. Modern theories suggest that coloring can release stress and promote better mental health. Perhaps the best thing about coloring for an adult with dyslexia—there are no words!

There are some hidden cognitive benefits to coloring as well: The act of putting pen or pencil to paper in a controlled manner improves brain function. You do not have to be working with text for this benefit. In addition, researchers have found that the task of staying within the lines can sharpen cognitive strengths.

To get the most benefit, utilize art-quality soft core colored pencils, gel pens, or water-based markers. The flexible pressure of applying quality pencils or markers to paper seems to add to the therapeutic benefits.

#3. Reframe Your Belief

BEST FOR: Examining negative feelings from a mature perspective

This strategy guides you in shifting the blame from yourself. It involves the power of perception. We might perceive that, for example, others have told us we were not smart. And they may have, but what resonates with us is our internal belief in what we were told.

There is power in reframing negative thoughts, challenging those unhealthy internal beliefs from a more mature perspective, by changing the way we interpret the events that spawned the view.

To do this, cognitive therapists recommend you:

1. Identify the predicament. For example, you were placed in the lowest reading group in grade school.
2. Analyze how it made you feel: embarrassed, inadequate.
3. Identify what thoughts the event recalls: "I'm stupid."
4. Regard the circumstances objectively: "I'm not stupid. My dyslexia made it difficult for me to learn to read, but I was good at other things."

The desirable outcome is to abandon the negative belief. Reframing takes conscious practice; you may have to revisit a deep-seated view from several angles before your perspective shifts. That's natural. If you feel stuck in a feeling of despair, please seek professional help.

#4. Broaden Your Mind

BEST FOR: Promoting positive self-worth

Audiobooks promote mental stimulation and emotional well-being, among countless additional benefits. Multiple studies have shown there is equal value in eye-reading and listening to audiobooks; both promote empathy, creativity, and a positive sense of self-worth. Exposure to literature allows one to experience how others face adversity, find solutions, and persevere. Also, books make us smarter!

Audiobooks allow access to stories and information that stimulate your intelligence. You are not limited to your reading level or reading speed. You are more likely to understand complex sentence structures. Natural pauses and emphasis will be evident when read by a proficient reader, making it easier to follow the story. And you might discover new vocabulary from words you may have passed over in eye-reading.

Moreover, audiobooks allow your brain to relax while promoting more productivity in menial tasks such as housework, driving, or walking. A wide variety of fiction and nonfiction books are available in audio format. Check with your public library; most offer free audiobooks that you can access on your phone or even a smartwatch!

#5. Stand Up and Move

BEST FOR: Boosting your mood and clearing your mind

This activity promotes physical and mental health. You do not have to have a rigorous exercise plan to reap medical and emotional benefits. In my experience, there is nothing like a walk outdoors: fresh air, sunshine, a wave or smile from a neighbor. In addition, walking allows our minds to wander, allowing for those ah-ha moments. A Stanford University study found that walking promoted divergent thinking, which led to creative outcomes, in 60 percent of the participants.

Walking can also boost your mood. Various studies have found that walking can override low feelings of sorrow or dread. However, keep in mind that another study emphasizes the importance of posture. When one concentrates on walking in an upright position, they experience significantly lower stress, less sleeplessness, and a marginal increase in feelings of empowerment compared with their slouching peers. Fascinating, isn't it? Experts generally agree as little as 15 minutes a day can provide physical and emotional benefits.

#6. Make Best Use of Your Constructive Mind

BEST FOR: Beginning your day

This strategy helps you make the best use of time when your mind is at its calmest.

For a while now, researchers have associated a healthy sleep cycle with creative thinking. More recent studies have focused on how healthy sleep positively impacts problem-solving. The theory is when we are in a deep sleep, our brain organizes information. When we enter the rapid eye movement (REM) stage of sleep, usually at the end of our sleep cycle, our brain discovers unexpected connections.

Your mind is in a light form of sleep as you transition to waking up every morning. Those waking moments can be crucial times to allow your brain to contemplate innovative ideas while you're still lying in bed. Try making the following practices part of your morning routine:

- Ask executive inquiring questions: What will I accomplish today? How will I prioritize my day? What can aid my focus and planning?

- Allow a few minutes to contemplate your thoughts before rushing out of bed.

- Take those still quiet moments to re-center and connect ideas while you have a calm mind.

#7. Create Margin in Your Day

BEST FOR: Calmness

This activity allows us to slow down and take time and enjoy the present.

The Theory of Margin, introduced in 1963 by educational psychology researcher Howard McClusky, measures the relationship of the load of life's events to the power to carry the load. McClusky theorized that as adults increase in age, so do their life stressors and demands, such as a career shift, raising children, or a spouse's death. Several daily factors are out of our control; thus, we must be prepared to meet the challenge of unpredictable crises. We need time to understand our circumstances and learn from and cope with changing events. Here are some principles to follow:

- Create margin in your daily routine by not overbooking. Modern expectations pressure us to schedule something for every second of the day. Allow blank space in your schedule so you can handle unexpected challenges and delays.

- Don't book everything back-to-back. Add 5 to 10 minutes breathing time between events.

- Designate 10 to 20 minutes to catch up with your spouse, partner, or children in the early evening. Of course, you can take longer than that, but if it's part of your schedule, you'll always have at least some time to connect on busy days.
- Allow yourself time to adjust, shift gears, and transition to new tasks.

Modern theories claim that adults who utilize margin with these strategies exhibit healthy motivation in pursuing self-improvement and education.

#8. Lift Your Mood with Music

BEST FOR: Inspiration

This strategy promotes a positive mindset. Various studies show that listening to music lowers stress, eases pain, improves mood, and provides comfort. Like audiobooks, music can accompany tedious tasks and be accessed on any device, including your phone.

Often, we listen to what we are familiar with, songs of our youth, or comfortable genres. Experts suggest we vary what music we listen to. We might try music today's teens enjoy, stimulating our brain to understand the new sound. Listening to songs from our past can bring us back to a pleasurable event, such as a first dance or kiss. Songs that focus on positive lyrics might lift our mood. Listen to your body; sometimes we need physical stimulation or mental inspiration; sometimes we just need a companion.

#9. Positive Thinking in Action

BEST FOR: Evoking positive emotions to build confidence and lower stress

This strategy suggests savoring a pleasant experience from your past. Think of how when eating a yummy dessert or five-star meal, we linger so we might appreciate the experience and allow it to enhance a positive feeling. Research suggests that savoring a positive moment has a positive effect on coping. Basically, you go to a happy time in your life to evoke positive emotions; you acknowledge and appreciate the enjoyable feelings—you reminisce. As a result, positive emotions help build confidence to handle the daily stressors in your life.

Psychologists suggest these steps:

1. Take the time to think about a happy event in your past—maybe a family trip or a visit to your grandparents' house.
2. Let the memory evoke whatever positive emotions come to mind—e.g., excitement, happiness, joy.
3. Visualize the details. In your mind's eye, try to generate detailed and moving images, with color and background.
4. Savor the emotions and the experience. Stay in the moment.
5. When the memory passes, focus on the pleasant feelings that remain. Meditate on your positive mental state.

Poring over photographs, listening to music from your past, or tasting childhood food from a happy time are other ways to reminisce. Be sure to keep this experience light and relaxing. If you feel you need help with intense past emotions, please seek professional therapy.

#10. Take a Mindful Moment

BEST FOR: Self-awareness and self-compassion

This strategy will relieve stress and refocus your thoughts. For example, you might find yourself overwhelmed by your workload, embarrassed by a snafu, or anxious about an upcoming event.

Mindfulness is the state or quality of focusing one's awareness on the present moment, without judgment. Mindfulness benefits include reduced stress and anxiety and improved sleep. Let's consider a hot cup of chamomile tea, for instance. You might enter a state of mindfulness with these steps:

1. Take a moment to feel the warm mug in your hand.
2. Take in the aroma.
3. Savor the moment.
4. Take a slow sip.
5. Let the apple-like taste linger in your mouth.
6. Enjoy the comfort of warm tea traversing your upper body.
7. Let out your "Aaah," exhaling a bit of steam.
8. Relish the delight of the moment.
9. If your awareness drifts away from the present, notice this, and gently bring your mind back to the sensations of the present moment.
10. Continue for as long as you like.

You can apply mindfulness to almost any activity—eating a savory or sweet snack, relaxing on a bench, taking a stroll through a park, even while sitting in a doctor's waiting room or standing in line at the supermarket.

Conclusion

As adults with dyslexia, often our biggest fear is that someone will discover our secret. It's difficult, but if we embrace dyslexia, we no longer have a secret; we are free to emphasize our strengths and continue to build on them. It is important to remember we cannot do it all—nobody can—but we can lean into our uniqueness to accomplish our goals.

In the next chapter, we will discuss how to improve your literacy skills. No matter how successful, each adult with dyslexia can improve to some extent on reading, spelling, or vocabulary. In fact, there is so much to learn about words! I look forward to exploring this with you.

CHAPTER 4

Improve Your Literacy Skills

Literacy is the ability to read and write. But a broader definition includes interpreting, creating, and computing information in print. So it's easy to see that literacy struggles can have a huge impact on someone's life. To understand how much dyslexia affects a particular person's literacy skills, we must evaluate the effort it takes that individual to decipher print. The core struggle with literacy for the individual with dyslexia happens at the word level, with shortcomings in reading, spelling, and pronouncing multisyllabic words. And that's where efforts to improve your literacy skills should focus. Scientific research has found that working to improve skills at the word level leads to exponential growth in the brain's ability to process language.

CARLA

Carla was a homeschool mom who came to me because she found reading to her children challenging. Even when reading children's books, she would stammer. Early on, Carla had been able to skip or even substitute for unfamiliar words. But lately her oldest, age seven, was beginning to catch her miscues. Carla wished to strengthen her oral reading ability.

    Carla began an Orton-Gillingham tutoring program (we'll explain what that is later in this chapter) to work on her decoding skills and oral reading fluency. At home, she practiced phonological awareness activities with her children. Carla also began reading books to herself before reading them out loud to her family. That way, she was familiar with the content and was able to work out any unknown words in advance.

> As Carla's oral reading improved, so did her confidence in reading to her children. She began teaching her children to read utilizing a scripted structured literacy curriculum. Over time, Carla learned reading skills alongside her kids. Carla reported that she still made mistakes, especially when she was tired. But reading out loud to her children was one of her favorite activities.

Dyslexic Adults Can Have a Variety of Literacy Challenges

Literacy generally refers to the ability to read, write, and solve math for everyday life functioning. It's applied knowledge that's connected to everything we do in our community. If your literacy isn't equal to the challenges of your life, you're not alone. According to the National Center for Education, the average reading level in the United States is below the eighth grade. And of those poor readers, approximately 70 to 80 percent are thought to have dyslexia.

Dyslexia doesn't mean your literacy is doomed to remain stunted. Many adults with dyslexia do become competent readers. In most cases, their development in reading was slower than their non-dyslexic peers, and they developed work-arounds. But frequently, their comprehension abilities are above average compared to their typical-reading peers.

Difficulty in reading is not as apparent in adults as it might be in children. Some bright adults with dyslexia struggle to read but are good at hiding their difficulties. Only the individual with dyslexia can gauge how hard or easy their own experience is in deciphering, understanding, and applying print to their real-time life. Each person's capability is unique. But we can identify some typical literacy challenges faced by people with dyslexia.

Decoding

Decoding, the ability to use letter-sound relationships to recognize a word, is an essential skill for effective reading. Without proper instruction, an adult with dyslexia will find it hard to interpret new words. If a reader is unable to decode an unfamiliar word, they are at a severe disadvantage in developing word identification skills. A history of poor decoding skills in childhood leads to slow reading speed in adulthood.

Reading Speed

Why are individuals with dyslexia slow readers? A dyslexic reader requires substantially more exposure to a word than their typical-reading peers before they can devote that word to memory. Also, in some people with dyslexia the brain takes longer to visually interpret symbols and transform them into a verbal output. So even if you recognize a word, it may take you longer to identify the word in your mind.

Reading Accuracy

Since the dyslexic brain does not automatically decode, it will substitute or skip over a word it does not quickly recognize. Sometimes words can be identified with other methods: The dyslexic brain can correctly guess the word by its context in the sentence or paragraph—for example that pony means "horse"—or replace the unknown word with a similar one. Or it may replace the unknown word with another one based on shape or size (reading lock as look) or beginning/ending sounds (reading component as complement), changing the meaning in the process. The dyslexic brain is always on the hunt for the big idea. So it's frustrating when words are read inaccurately in text and the confused reader must reread something several times to grasp the meaning.

Reading Comprehension

In people who have dyslexia, brain strengths in big picture thinking, analytical skills, and detecting patterns lead to deep comprehension abilities. Attention and interest are intricately connected to comprehension in all readers, but especially with people who have dyslexia. For beginning readers, the strengths of dyslexia can compensate for the difficulties. When I assess a third grader's oral reading, it is not uncommon for the student with dyslexia to make several mistakes but have a deep and accurate understanding of the passage based on contextual cues. However, in adolescence and adulthood, the reading material becomes more complex, and there are fewer pictures. The individual can no longer rely simply on context to understand the text that they can't decode.

Reading Aloud

Reading aloud requires a high level of vocabulary and visual-spatial integration. The reader must decipher the print, use their word knowledge to make sense of meaning and grammar, and then express that word with the correct tone for syntax, all while detecting the placement of the word in the sentence for pausing. When a person with dyslexia reads aloud, they make the mistakes that they've gotten used to in silent reading, resulting in skipping or substituting words. Along with that, their oral reading will display unnatural pauses in sentences. It's no wonder that individuals with dyslexia sidestep reading aloud since it exposes the deficits that they're trying to keep secret.

Learning a Foreign Language

Learning a foreign language in an academic setting is typically torturous for someone with dyslexia. Language students are expected to read and write and in most cases must participate in informal conversations to progress beyond the beginner level. While someone with dyslexia might be limited to learning a foreign language at the basic level of reading and writing, this capacity varies. Some of my students who had to fulfill a graduation requirement have found online courses or American Sign Language classes to be passable. And some of my more analytical students have enjoyed learning Latin.

Helpful Technology for Dyslexic Readers

Technology allows those of us who have dyslexia to lean into our cognitive strengths. And using technology in today's workplace has become common for everyone. Here's an overview of the possibilities; please refer to the Resources section for recommended technical tools.

Audiobooks and digital books provide access to higher-level thinking, complex sentence structure, and new vocabulary that a person with dyslexia would find challenging in print. In addition, digital books offer the ability to immediately look up a word for meaning and pronunciation.

Reading applications for web and PDF files are readily available. Many digital devices and apps have these read-aloud functions built in. Most reading apps use text-to-speech software that only works on web pages, PDF, and word processing applications. But optical character recognition (OCR) systems allow one to scan a printed document and hear it read out loud. There are even several reading pens on the market, which scan lines of text and read them aloud.

Writing applications are a must these days. I suggest filtering your polished work through your word processor's embedded spelling and grammar features, then using a separate application to provide a different perspective. Always have what you wrote read back to you. Most processors have a read-back function under the review tab. Software with advanced functions to help with writing continues to advance; some even give you occasional updates on how your writing is improving.

It's Never Too Late to Improve Your Reading

You may have found a work-around to avoid or minimize the reading you need to do, or you may be an avid reader. In my experience, most adults with dyslexia continue to feel burdened with how difficult it is to read aloud, no matter their age or accomplishments.

There's every reason to try to lighten that burden. Studies have shown that when given an opportunity to learn, individuals with dyslexia have tremendous perseverance. Many adults with dyslexia are not able to reach their potential because of continued difficulty in reading. You might be trying to improve, aware that something is holding you back, but not making progress. Because you do not know what efficient reading feels like, you may not recognize the need to improve your word-level reading. Some people with dyslexia believe their problem lies in comprehension and fluency, but these are indicators, not typically the cause, of a reading struggle.

Have you given up on making things better? Don't. It is never too late to enhance your reading abilities. It is essential to explore the sound and structure of words. A widely recognized, age-old approach to teaching reading is known as Orton-Gillingham. Let's take a look.

The Orton-Gillingham Approach

The Orton-Gillingham method is a highly structured, researched-based approach that's designed to break words down into their smallest parts and then build them back up to a cohesive whole. Designed by researchers and educators Samuel Orton and Anna Gillingham nearly 100 years ago, Orton-Gillingham was the first learning program designed specifically for struggling readers. Orton-Gillingham, which mimics the natural ways that children learn to read, is considered the gold standard for teaching students with dyslexia. The primary goal is word-level reading, not comprehension. Several contemporary curricula are based on it. The basis of Orton-Gillingham curricula is to:

- Eliminate the need for a person to memorize almost all words
- Simultaneously introduce decoding and spelling skills
- Expand decoding methods beyond sounding out a word
- Emphasize understanding the "how" and "why" behind reading and spelling

- Focus on word-level reading with continuous student-teacher interaction

In any Orton-Gillingham curriculum, there's a clear connection between symbols—letters and letter combinations—and the sounds they represent. The goal of building this awareness is embedded throughout the program. Orton-Gillingham programs are systematic, requiring each lesson to build on the previous. Every student starts from the beginning; nothing is assumed about their reading ability. Because Orton-Gillingham operates on diagnostic assessment, the pace is determined by the student's need.

What Is Phonological Awareness?

As we discussed back in chapter 1, phonological awareness is a part of phonological processing. It is a foundational skill needed to decode and spell words. Phonological awareness is the ability to hear and manipulate the separate elements that make up a word, syllable, rhyme, or initial sound. Referred to as phonemes, these sounds are the smallest elements of spoken or written language. The dyslexic brain finds it exceedingly difficult to break information or sounds into these smaller parts. Persons with dyslexia sometimes cannot even hear these distinct sounds. They know that a word is spelled with individual letters, but cannot easily isolate, manipulate, and sequence the phonemes that the letters represent.

Weak phonological awareness is a hallmark indicator of untreated dyslexia. Adults who lack phonological awareness have been blocked from becoming efficient readers. It's hard to correct this problem on your own, because usually we can't perceive the impact that weak phonological awareness has on our reading and word comprehension. There is good news: Phonological awareness is responsive to strategic instruction and practice. It's never too late to improve this ability.

How Does It Show Up in Adults?

Weak phonological processing is evident in adults through speech and spelling. An adult with poor phonological awareness may transpose sound properties in words they spell or say. For example, try spelling the word dyslexia. Despite spelling dyslexia a million times, I still transpose letters if I do not give it my full concentration when I'm writing or typing it. The same is true in speech. Adults with phonological weakness will inevitably mispronounce, or avoid saying, certain words when recalling a multisyllabic word.

When to Seek Help with Literacy

As an adult with dyslexia, you will absolutely benefit from expanding your knowledge of word structure, improving your decoding skills, learning spelling patterns, and working on your writing style and structure. But to make progress, you must follow a systematic approach to learning these things. I offer many options in the Resources.

Where to start? If you suspect your reading skills are below a proficient level for your daily life, I suggest seeking a dyslexia specialist for explicit reading and spelling instruction, using an Orton-Gillingham system. Adults below a proficient reading level might attend a community literacy program through their local library or adult learning centers. Online adult reading programs are also available.

There are no quick fixes—you'll have to put in the work. But it's worth it.

Literacy Encompasses a Range of Skills

If you've resigned yourself to not reading except when necessary, keep in mind that the definition of literacy goes beyond the ability to read and write. Literacy includes interpreting, creating, and computing information in print. All of these are core challenges for a person with dyslexia. Although dyslexia is linked to reading, there is so much more to its impact on literary skills, the skills you need in everyday life. Here are some of the capabilities that are strengthened when you bolster your literacy skills. We'll look at specific skill-boosting strategies at the end of this chapter.

Spelling

There are various ways to improve your spelling, but memorization is rarely one of them. While we can commit several words to memory, our long-term memory is limited. Likewise, even though we love patterns, that's not always enough to spell a word correctly. Knowing the reason behind a word's spelling encourages broader spelling skills. And there are fewer essential rules to spelling than you might think. In addition to knowing the rules, you can learn to look for word parts and find related words, like explode and explosion. These can often assist in the intricacies of spelling longer, more complicated words.

Vocabulary

Developing your vocabulary is vital to developing literacy. Vocabulary aids our word recognition in print. It expands our minds to new concepts and relationships in words. Also, developing a rich vocabulary just makes you seem smarter! I suggest you spend quality time reading and do not skip over unknown words. I appreciate that you cannot do this extra work with everything that you read. Nonetheless, I propose you approach new words with an inquiring mindset as much as possible.

Reading Fluency

The only way to become fluent is to practice. But in order to practice good reading habits, you need to read material that won't require you to guess at the words. I suggest trying well-regarded youth or young adult novels, like The Giver by Lois Lowry or Where the Red Fern Grows by Wilson Rawls. There are countless examples of quality young adult (YA) literature out there; much of it, I venture to bet, you have not read. These books offer complex sentence structure, vocabulary, and strong literary elements. Plus, they are fun to read, often offering positive outcomes to life's complications.

Reading Comprehension

Whenever you're able, before you start reading something, take some time to know what you are reading, the purpose you're reading it for, and what you expect to gain from the text. I also suggest recapping what you're reading at logical stopping points, like paragraphs, sections, and chapters, pausing to check your knowledge of key ideas. As you read, connect the content to something you already know. Evoke your sensory system to visualize images; make a movie in your head as the information or story progresses.

Practice, Practice, Practice!

Whichever area of literacy you would like to improve, you will need to practice. Practicing a new skill enhances our overall brain processing and working memory. Just as muscles get stronger with exercise, our brain becomes smarter as we challenge it. If done with intention and a drive to improve, the skills we practice become more automatic with time. And when you master one level or skill, it frees up some brain power for you to work on another.

Strategies to Improve Your Literacy

It's time to put what you've learned about literacy into action. Remember that these 10 strategies are intended to enhance your skill, not overwhelm you. Read through them and use those you feel are relevant to your progress. You can always come back and try others as they fit in with your journey.

#1. Take Up Word Watching
BEST FOR: **Enhancing your vocabulary**

A fun way to enhance your vocabulary is to build a collection of unique and challenging words. Bird watchers keep a list of notable birds that they see in the wild; you can become a word watcher and make a record of intriguing words that you come across in everyday life.

Start keeping a digital or written word bank containing your favorite words, so you can review them and try them out. When you encounter unfamiliar words while reading, type them into your phone or a convenient device and look up the definition. Think about the word and try to picture its meaning, invoking your senses. One trick to remembering a new word is to associate it with a related familiar word. For example, melodious—musically pleasant—relates to melody, a quality of music.

Begin using new words in writing before trying them in conversation. Your visual image of the word might aid in saying it correctly. If you are unsure how to use a word, a simple internet search like "how to use [word] in a sentence" can often yield your answer. Don't be afraid to use new words in your writing. Tools like grammar check can help you screen your usage if you're feeling unsure.

#2. Learn the Rules for Syllable Division

BEST FOR: Reading speed and efficiency

This activity will aid you in reading multisyllabic words quickly by pointing out how to divide words effortlessly.

There are dependable patterns to how word syllables fit together. Knowing where to divide a word can help with sounding out vowels, which makes it easier to accurately identify words. These patterns can help you pronounce an unfamiliar word and begin to recognize it in context.

Study the following rules for how words are divided into their syllables:

- When vowels occur in pairs, like ai, oo, or ea (raining, footwear, beacon), these vowel teams are not separated: rai-ning, foot-wear, bea-con.

- When there is only one consonant between two vowels, the consonant most often goes to the back part of the word. So, bonus is bo-nus; tomato is to-ma-to.
- When there are two consonants between vowels, separate the consonants most of the time. So napkin is nap-kin; splendid is splen-did. The exception is to keep common blends together.
- A vowel only needs one consonant after it to close off the syllable. The other consonants will usually go to the second half of the word. For example, complex is com-plex, not comp-lex. And subscript is sub-script.
- Divide compound words—that is words made up of smaller words—into their component words, like sand-box, lady-bug, hair-pin.
- The letter y is a vowel most of the time; it is only used as a consonant at the beginning of a word, like yellow, or a syllable, like canyon (divided as can-yon, since y is the second consonant between vowels).

#3. Practice Prosody

BEST FOR: Improving oral reading

This strategy, based on Susan Barton's popular technique, helps with oral reading fluency, silent reading comprehension, and reading speed.

Prosody is the stress and intonation used in oral reading, including pauses. People with dyslexia do not readily know when to pause within a sentence when they're reading aloud.

Just like words can be broken into phonemes, sentences can be split into phrases, or sentence parts. Each phrase plays a role in the sentence: who/what, did what, where, when, why, how.

For instance, consider this sentence: The elephant jumped over the tree because he was scared.

The "what" phrase is The elephant; the "did what" is jumped; "where?" is over the tree; and "why?" is because he was scared. Note that most "where" and "when" phrases begin with a preposition: "in the house," "after dinner."

It's not an exact science, but pausing between these phrases usually makes for good prosody. Begin by identifying phrases, and using them to pause while reading aloud, in simple sentences at your easy reading level. For instance, these lines taken from My Father's Dragon, a 1948 children's book by Ruth Stiles Gannett, are divided at meaningful pauses for natural fluency.

That very afternoon / my father and Cat / went down to the docks / to see about ships / going to the island of Tangerine.

They found out / that a ship / would be sailing / next week.

Read them aloud to see how it sounds when you pause between phrases.

#4. Broaden Your Reading List

BEST FOR: **Practicing print reading and developing a general love for literature**

Everyone should expand the breadth of their reading. Along with trying out new authors and subject matter, mix up the formats. Print books will help you develop important mechanical reading skills, while audiobooks will allow you to take on more ambitious books that challenge your mind and develop your intellect.

To practice fluency, which means reading at a comfortable pace with accuracy, it's imperative to read at a manageable level. For this purpose, choose material you can read without needing to guess or skip over words so you can gradually build your skills at a comfortable level.

To improve your word-reading skills—that is, to get better at accurately identifying words in text—I suggest choosing content that requires greater concentration to read. You should be able to identify most of the words in the text, but not all of them. Slow down and notice words and sentence structure. Look up the meaning and pronunciation of words you do not recognize. Make a note of clever sentence structures. Use an e-reader with text-to-voice and dictionary functions for help when needed.

Most importantly, read what interests you in the genre you prefer, whether it's novels, news articles, nonfiction, self-help, biographies, or whatever's appealing. Make a reasonable goal, perhaps starting with 10 to 30 minutes of reading per day.

Simultaneously keeping up with an audiobook at your listening level will allow you to enjoy advanced texts. Individuals with dyslexia tend to have a higher listening comprehension level than reading level.

#5. Learn the Rules of Spelling

BEST FOR: Improving spelling skills and learning word origins

Learning the why and how of spelling brings tremendous benefits to literacy. As it turns out, most words are spelled the way they are for a reason. If we activate our brain to learn these rules behind the spelling, we expand our spelling skills exponentially. And it might surprise you how few spelling rules are needed to be a good speller.

Here are a few simple rules to get you started:

- Double the consonants at the end of a word with one vowel and that ends in f, l, or s (as in gruff, skill, or kiss).

- You only write -ck, -tch, or -dge immediately after a short vowel (examples: back, batch, badge).

- The digraph ch sounds like /ch/ in American words (chess), /k/ in words of Greek origin (orchid), and /sh/ in words that originated in French (chef). It's not always easy for someone with dyslexia to distinguish between sounds like this in speech. Someone who has dyslexia might hear a /chr/ sound at the beginning of a word a word like train, instead of /tr/.

And that's just the tip of the iceberg! Use your inquiring mind to learn how and why a word is spelled, and you'll enter a fascinating world of history and language. Books, guides, and internet searches are readily available to help you navigate.

#6. Memorize Problem Words

BEST FOR: Learning words that don't follow the rules

Some words don't fit into established patterns and are best memorized. This includes many commonly used words like because or doubt.

Mnemonics can help. For example, to remember how to spell because I teach:

Big Elephants Can't Always Understand Small Elephants

This catchy phrase is easier to recall than the random letters, especially for people with dyslexia. Try creating your own memorable phrases to remember the spelling of words that you struggle with.

Another helpful tactic is to relate a challenging word to a familiar one. As an example, we can remember how to spell doubt by considering its relationship to the word double.

"If you doubt something, you think about it twice—double."

In that way, a word that we know how to spell becomes a guide to a more difficult word with similar spelling.

A third option is to create a sequence using imagery that you can see in your mind's eye.

If you want to learn the spelling of Mississippi, you might close your eyes and repeat the spelling aloud while visualizing each letter. The next time you have to spell it, try recalling that sequence of images.

#7. Try Structured Word Inquiry

BEST FOR: Learning to spell words by their construction

This strategy will encourage you to gain a deeper knowledge of word structures and word origins. A word's derivatives and origin impact how we spell it and its meaning.

The term structured word inquiry (SWI) was coined by researcher Peter Bowers, founder of the WordWorks Literacy Centre in Ontario, Canada, to describe the process of understanding word origins and meanings. SWI investigates how a word is structured and its relationship to other words.

For example, the word does is typically taught as an irregular word. But by investigating the base word, do, we find that spelling represents the metamorphosis of the word in a familiar pattern, though the pronunciation doesn't reflect that. Do becomes does the way that go becomes goes.

That answers a spelling question, but we can also use structured word inquiry to build an extensive vocabulary. For example, using the Latin base pend (to hang), I can create all the following words by adding prefixes and suffixes. By knowing how words are built, one is better able to understand their meaning and spelling.

sus + pend + ed → suspended

im + pend + ing → impending

ex + pend + s → expends

ap + pend + ix → appendix

de + pend + able → dependable

There's a lot more information available about SWI. Structured word inquiry can be used with Latin roots, Greek word parts, or traditional base words. You can find some more information in the Resources.

#8. Read with Purpose

BEST FOR: Comprehension of textbooks, news articles, and publications

This strategy will aid you in comprehending large informational texts and info-dense documents.

When grappling with factual articles or data-filled publications, taking a more strategic approach than simply reading from beginning to end can be helpful.

1. Identify the topic of the document. Often the title will give it away, but not always. You may need to scan a short section to pinpoint

repeated words and ideas. Typically, the topic will be evident within the first few paragraphs; also, it's usually reflected in the last paragraph.

2. Identify what you already know about the subject at hand.
3. Ask yourself: What do I want to learn about this?
4. As you read, make a note of any key points that interest you, add to your knowledge, or are essential to the topic.
5. Afterward, take a few seconds to summarize what you read; say it aloud to accentuate your ability to later recall the details.

If the material is difficult, you might simplify the text as you read by highlighting essential details, streamlining the information. Some reading comprehension applications offer features to simplify the text. For example, many web browsers offer a reading view to clear distractions from web pages. Reading applications like Read&Write literacy software allow the reader to highlight text in different colors, categorizing the information in a separate document.

#9. Find the Story

BEST FOR: Improving comprehension of what you read

Deep comprehension of a story requires a great deal of working memory and the skill to sequence events. One way to follow a story and understand its elements is to document the rise and fall of the action, climax, and resolution. If you're having trouble following a story, biography, or history, try to outline the plot as if it were a fairytale. Creating this type of synopsis works well to narrow the content to its most significant elements.

As a model, these are my notes taken from a summary of The Adventures of Pinocchio on Britannica.com.

Characters (this can also include the setting and time period)

- Geppetto: Wanted a child

- Pinocchio: G's abused creation, who runs away
- Fox and Cat: Lure and steal from Pinocchio

Rise and fall of action

- Fox and Cat hang Pinocchio
- Fairy saves Pinocchio
- Pinocchio lies to Fairy; nose grows
- Pinocchio tricked again by Fox and Cat
- 2x Pinocchio tried to attend school, 2x led astray; turns into a donkey

Climax and resolution

- Pinocchio swallowed by a shark
- Pinocchio finds Geppetto in shark's belly
- Caring for Geppetto, Pinocchio turns into a real boy

Once you have practiced recognizing plot elements in easier, shorter stories, you will start recognizing them in longer texts.

#10. Use Technology to Your Advantage

BEST FOR: Promoting efficiency and supporting your reading

Over the years, my clients have shared many tips and tricks for utilizing technology to manage dyslexia. Here are two of the most helpful tools.

Let's talk more about utilizing e-readers and tablets to read. Novels, news articles, and magazines are all available in digital form. E-readers and devices offer a multitude of accessories. You can choose text background and letter color. Text font, size, and spacing can be customized. Most text-to-voice functions highlight the corresponding words; some bring the line being read to the forefront. Others utilize a strip to isolate the line being read. Some browsers and applications can simplify the text by eliminating any excess information not needed for comprehension. Explore all the options available and take full advantage of the ones that help you.

The best advice I can pass on to you as a general audience of adults with dyslexia is to always have your written communications read back to you. Find a text-to-voice editing function you like, one that has correct pausing and sounds as natural as possible. My favorite read-back option is Microsoft Word 365's "Read Aloud" function. When I use it, inevitably I'm surprised by how many mistakes I made. When I read my words back to myself, I don't catch my errors, because I remember what I intended to write instead of seeing where I went wrong.

Conclusion

Science continues to illuminate the reading brain. As an adult with dyslexia, there is no doubt you have already shown remarkable grit. That tenacity will serve you well. Although there is no quick solution to improving your literacy skills, you can enhance your skills over time by maintaining an inquiring growth mindset. Continue to follow your interest in language skills with the confidence that although reading and spelling have been difficult in the past, you can better understand the elements of language. You may even find your passion in the process.

In the next chapter, we will continue to explore the complex reading brain. The language brain requires auditory and visual information to recognize print. Where do these modalities fit in the conceptual web of dyslexia?

CHAPTER 5

Sharpen Your Auditory, Visual, and Spatial Skills

The reading brain is a complex system that relies on integrating both auditory and visual information. Dyslexia is not a problem with hearing or vision; in other words, a hearing aid or eyeglasses will not help issues revolving around dyslexia. But it does impose both strengths and challenges involving the way that our sight and hearing work together in the reading process.

> ## STERLING
>
> As an operations coordinator in a manufacturing plant, each morning Sterling must present announcements to his group of 10 to 15 workers. Sterling reports this being a terrifying chore. He has to practice extensively and write out everything he wants to say. If he tries to just wing it, he stumbles and skips over words he's unsure of pronouncing.
>
> Sterling reports being a good listener but speaking can be problematic. He cannot recall the words to say or how to pronounce them. Sterling uses simple words to get his point across. He uses technology to figure out the pronunciation of words, then practices them over and over again. Sometimes his wife helps.
>
> When Sterling sought help at age 36, he discovered that he had weak phonological processing. He could not identify the sounds that made up words or their sequence. Sterling began instruction in phonemic sequencing three times a week.
>
> After a few months, words were beginning to make more sense to him. Soon Sterling was able to drop his sessions to one day a week of tutoring with some activities at home. Although he feels more

> comfortable in his speaking role, Sterling knows he has a way to go. One of his motivating factors is his young daughter. One day, he wants to be able to help her with her homework.

Auditory, Visual, and Spatial Skills in a Dyslexic Individual

How one learns differs among all persons, including people with dyslexia. But there are commonalities. We all use auditory and visual channels to receive, understand, and retain information. Our spatial abilities combine with visual skills, enabling us to read and write. Whatever our particular strengths, an extensive integration process goes on between these sensory channels when we read. Our auditory perception takes in the information for phonological awareness, while visual and spatial processing must make sense of the connections.

High intellect typically cannot mask auditory, visual, or spatial weaknesses. But these are not the most important attributes of dyslexia. It's important to remember that dyslexia is distinguished by a different way that the brain processes language.

True to the dual nature of dyslexia, people can have significant differences between strengths and weaknesses relating to these three senses. For example, listening comprehension is typically a strength with dyslexia, yet phonological awareness—also an auditory skill—tends to be a weakness. Strong visual-spatial capabilities allow many people with dyslexia the gift of imagining objects from multiple angles. Still, these same individuals might struggle with mirror imaging of letters when trying to read printed text.

Auditory Perception and Discrimination Challenges

There's no denying that our first exposure to language is affected by what we hear. Our earliest experiences form a foundation of how we perceive language and discriminate sounds. If our interpretation is faulty, learning to read and spell will be challenging. If this problem goes unrecognized, it will continue to impact every aspect of a person's literacy.

Dyslexia stems from weak phonological processing. This includes auditory perception, how the brain recognizes and uses information that it receives via hearing. Dyslexic brains prefer to gather the overall gist of a situation, paying less attention to perceiving the smaller components of language and their correct sequence.

Auditory discrimination, the brain's ability to distinguish between similar sounds, can also be affected by weak phonological processing. Someone with poor auditory discrimination might have difficulty distinguishing words with genuinely similar sounds, especially short vowel sounds in unaccented syllables. Letter sounds that use similar mouth movement, like the sound of /f/ and /th/, can be problematic to differentiate. Likewise, someone challenged in auditory discrimination will have a challenging time repeating complex words. For example, ask someone to say a word like mischievous to you. See if you can repeat the word 10 times without looking at it in print.

Phonological Memory

The essence of phonological memory is the coding of bits of language for temporary storage in working memory. This complex process involves the brain holding on to speech for a microsecond to enable repeating that data aloud with precise articulation. When this process is inefficient, retaining longer words and sentences in working memory becomes taxing. Phonological memory weakness is not as noticeable in early reading skills. It's more often apparent after third grade, when the words and sentences in reading assignments become longer.

Phonological Sequencing

Phonemes, as we discussed in chapter 4, are the most minor units of sound. For example, the sounds represented by the letter b and the diagraph (two letter symbol) ch are phonemes. They make one sound when placed in a sequence of other sounds to create a syllable. When the brain hears a word or syllable, it must distinguish the series in which these phonemes occur in order to correctly reproduce the word or syllable. If the brain can't hold the sounds in sequence, the result will be transposed or omitted phonemes. Hence, phonological sequencing is essential to word identification, spelling, and speaking.

Visual Perception and Discrimination Challenges

Visual perception is the brain's ability to understand what the eyes see. Likewise, visual discrimination is the brain's ability to match or differentiate between two symbols or images. Once the brain visually takes in letters, words, and numbers, they are processed in the language area of the brain to attach meaning. Since dyslexia makes processing language difficult, this information can be distorted, impacting reading, handwriting, spelling, and even math.

Other common challenges involving visual perception and discrimination include:

- Copying information from near and far sources, like from a textbook and an information board
- Not noticing errors in writing
- Mixing print and cursive letters in handwriting
- Problems distinguishing similarly shaped and sized words
- Reversing of letters and numbers
- Reading a word as its mirror image, like was for saw
- Omission or transposition of letters, numbers, or words
- Difficulty recalling sequences of words or letters

Visual perception can be broken up into several skills. Let's examine those which are most relevant to people with dyslexia. It should be noted, though, that not all people with dyslexia will have weaknesses in visual perception. And in those that do, abilities will vary.

Visual Closure

Visual closure is the skill of identifying a form that is not entirely represented. This skill involves abstract problem-solving, which is a gift of dyslexia. Recently, I had an online student read a sentence that was only partly visible. He could read the sentence without error just by seeing the top third of each letter. And yet this same student tends to guess incorrectly in his typical reading.

Visual Perception Affects Math

Numbers can be complex for people with dyslexia to work with. For example, visual discrimination influences how we attend to details and identify distinctions in size, shape, orientation, and sequence. Likewise, visual memory affects how we recall an image.

Do you remember learning long division in upper elementary school? We were supposed to follow sequential steps on paper and visually attend to the direction in which to divide, multiply, subtract, place, and bring down the numbers.

Then came algebra, full of new language and symbols. For people with dyslexia, math errors might be blamed on carelessness, when visual perception may be the culprit.

Visual Form Consistency

Visual form consistency is the ability to recognize identical forms and distinguish between forms of different sizes, shapes, or orientations, like the letters b and d, or b and p. With visual form consistency, you can distinguish a symbol based on its shape alone, regardless of orientation.

Visual Memory

This capability is the ability to recall specific details of a given symbol, image, or shape after a short pause and then identify it within a set of similar forms. Someone with untreated dyslexia might be able to recall objects or images. But they might have a significantly more challenging time remembering the details of a word, number, or sentence, even within seconds of viewing it.

Visual Sequential Memory

With good visual sequential memory, you can recall and reproduce a series of images in the correct sequence after viewing them. The sequence can be stored in long-term memory. For instance, this ability allows you to know that g comes before h without needing to sing the alphabet song. Visual sequential memory often presents challenges in adults with dyslexia, at least to some degree.

Spatial Awareness

Spatial awareness is the ability to determine one's current orientation in space and time. Without it, reading a map or directions in a new city can be complicated, which is why people with dyslexia often navigate using landmarks and familiar objects in their environment. For those of us with dyslexia, following a GPS app when walking can be hilarious. The app says head east, and we head west. It might take several steps until you understand that you went the wrong way.

I was once driving in Peoria, just north of Phoenix, Arizona. Hills sprouted up everywhere. Near my home in Northern California, I was used to using the mountains on one side and the ocean on the other to get a sense of direction. No matter how hard I tried, I never did navigate myself in Peoria. I was very much dependent on Google Maps.

Adults with dyslexia may confuse left and right. During times of exhaustion, they may even write a letter or number backward. Problems with placing words on paper or word size can indicate spatial challenges. Fortunately, spatial awareness is all about our relationship to the environment, which people with dyslexia excel at.

Spatial Orientation and Spatial Perception

Spatial orientation is the ability to perceive our position in relation to an object. Spatial perception is our ability to interpret the shape, space, and location of objects around us and anticipate their movement. Spatial perception comes into play with nonverbal language like facial expressions and for conceiving three-dimensional imagery. Both are essential for perceiving our position in our environment and for allowing us to see other points of view and anticipate change. Together, they provide information that enables us to move through the world and are typically strengths for folks with dyslexia.

Many Dyslexics Have Inherently Good Spatial Awareness

Someone with dyslexia naturally understands their environment. They can envision how things interact from different perspectives. Imagine holding a mug. Can you picture looking down at the mug, at the back, the front, or underneath? This task is simple for a person with high visual-spatial reasoning, but not easy for a more pragmatic thinker. Strong spatial awareness also promotes out-of-the-box thinking, problem-solving, and new ideas. This ability to see multiple angles is why dyslexics are heavily represented in careers like entrepreneurs, inventors, athletes, and so much more.

Remember, Everyone Is Different

Dyslexics are not any different from the general population in that they have distinct learning preferences and strengths. You may have one or more of the challenges discussed in this chapter. However, the dual nature of dyslexia suggests you might have an opposing strength related to that challenge. You may have difficulty with two-dimensional images on a page, for example, but be excellent at designing an object in your head. You may not be able to follow a street map, maybe you even get lost with Google Maps, but you can navigate your city with ease using landmarks and memory. You may have incredible listening comprehension but not be able to hear isolated sounds in words. Whatever the give-and-take is, you are unique.

Strategies to Improve Your Auditory, Visual, and Spatial Skills

This chapter's strategies are intended to assist in managing visual and auditory perception issues associated with dyslexia. Don't feel pressured to use them all; review the list and try the ones that seem most relevant to your situation.

#1. Be a Purposeful Listener

BEST FOR: Improving auditory perception and discrimination

This strategy trains you for actively listening to the words you hear in conversation or during the course of your day. You must activate your working memory to listen intently and hear distinct elements in our language.

One way to build this habit is to listen to a song and try to recall and repeat the words. I once lived overseas and belonged to a group of young multicultural moms from different countries whose common language was English. I was the only American English first-language speaker in the group, so my friends tasked me to explain words in popular American rock songs. (This was before you could just search online for song lyrics.) I had not realized until then that I did not really listen to the words of songs. I knew the gist of what a song was about, but distinguishing each word was a chore. Often the other women in the group could better distinguish a word than I could. They would pronounce the word, then I would define it. We made a good team!

You can use the same approach with a poem or podcast. Have a poem read aloud to you. Try to repeat one line at a time, working up to a couplet and eventually a stanza or verse.

Listen to a podcast or webinar that offers a high vocabulary level in a subject you are familiar with or even an expert on. Pause and relisten to complex words, phrases, and sentence structures. Try to repeat the excerpts as if you were practicing a new language. In some ways, that's what you are doing.

#2. Develop Your Working Memory

BEST FOR: **Expanding your working memory for reading**

Experts believe that repetitive practice, or drilling, can expand one's ability to apply new information automatically. In other words, if you practice a new skill repeatedly in a drill format, you will be able to fall back on that skill under pressure when you need it.

Think about the soccer players we mentioned in chapter 2. To learn to make a corner shot, they have to practice over and over, countless times, in a controlled setting. With outside instruction from a coach or peer, they continually improve their technique. Eventually the player can make that shot during games, with few misses. You can challenge your reading brain the same way.

Suppose you tend to misread words in print. In that case, you might practice reading a list of genuinely alike words: discourse, disclose, displease, displeasure, disappoint, disappointment.

If you cannot sustain attention while you read, you might set a timer to track how long you can read before your attention wanders. Begin expanding the time by one or two minutes with each drill.

#3. Listen to Spell

BEST FOR: **Breaking down sounds for spelling**

There is a relationship between what we hear and how we spell. Most of that connection is developed before we learn to read. However, it's never too late to identify a sound-symbol relationship.

Try this process with a few words that you have trouble spelling, which have two or more syllables in them:

First, identify how many syllables the word has by how many times your chin drops when you pronounce it. For instance, the word dyslexia has four syllables, dys-lex-i-a. The number of syllables is not dependent on word size. The word complicate has only three syllables.

Next, break down the sounds within each syllable. What sounds do you hear? What letters spell the sound?

Sometimes there's more than one way to spell the same sound, like vowel sounds and some consonants, such as /g/ and /k/ sounds. Similarly, in the word ambiguous, -ous says /us/, the o is silent. Nonetheless, by isolating the smaller parts that make up more complex words, you have a better chance of at least getting the spelling close enough for spellcheck to register. You might also notice patterns of related words, sparking an interest to learn more about their relationship.

#4. Phonemic Awareness

BEST FOR: Refining your phonological processing

A key to improving phonological awareness is to listen to specific qualities of words and phrases, rather than only paying attention to the gist of a communication. These activities will develop intentional listening skills in everyday scenarios.

Listen to the details in words you know. Learn to articulate with excellence by noticing each phoneme within a word. Look up how to pronounce the word on a web browser; listen to the pronunciation and slow it down if possible.

Break words apart. Become familiar with the number of syllables in a word. Find what vowel sound glues each syllable together.

Learn to recognize consonant blends. These are two or three consonants spoken together, each making their own sound. Often dyslexia makes it tough to hear each distinct sound. Try writing out words and using color markers to represent the sounds that make up the syllables.

Practice these phonological awareness activities with the young people in your life. Promoting phonological awareness in the early stages of learning language, through first grade, will improve anyone's reading skills over their lifetime.

This list is not inclusive. Look for other ways to become more aware of the slightest sounds or phonemes in your life.

#5. Feel the Sound

BEST FOR: Activating phonological awareness

This strategy is focused on sensory feedback coming from identifying individual phonemes, the smallest units of sound. There is a physical movement of our lips or tongue when we say consonant sounds. These sounds require specific mouth actions.

There are speech apps available for Apple and Android operating systems that display the associated oral-motor action for a word. I use Speech Tutor. The premise is that seeing the action helps you relate the phoneme to its written symbol. Knowing how the mouth moves to make the sounds helps you distinguish the differences.

For example, consider the sound of the letter t. Can you feel your tongue tap? Sound the letter p. Do you feel your lips pop open? Remembering these oral motor sensations is important in helping you distinguish phonemes.

Some letter pairs evoke a similar sensation or feel. Try articulating the sounds of these letters:

p and b

k and g

t and d

f and v

s and z

ch (as in chair) and j

n and r

For each pair, try to identify the similarities in how your mouth or tongue moves and how you use your breath.

#6. Completing a Picture

BEST FOR: Promoting orthographic skills in a two-dimensional drawing

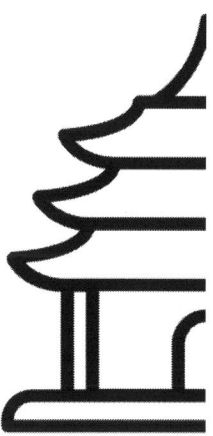

This activity will evoke visual perception and spatial awareness. This is especially helpful for those who have weak visual closure. Part of an image is provided here; complete the picture by adding the missing lines or duplicating the image.

Continue to practice with black and white two-dimensional images of your choice. Print them out and fold the image in half. Secure the folded paper onto another blank sheet. Then, sketch the missing side to complete the form.

#7. Drawing/Art

BEST FOR: Encouraging visual-spatial organization

This strategy will engage your creative side. Did you know that, as an artist, you are manipulating spatial organization? It's true. In color art, a painter controls the contrast between colors; a sketcher or sculptor assimilates shapes and location. These are all ways for an artist to organize space according to their preferences.

Some of you are creative; your dyslexic gifts may enable you to picture a detailed drawing in your mind. Find your medium, whether it's a traditional one like painting or pencil sketching, a three-dimensional format like sculpture or ceramics, or a modern digital or video app. Joining a community class might be an excellent place to start.

For those not confident in their skills, digital art apps might offer a bridge between technical and creative ability, allowing more access to your imagination.

#8. Solving Jigsaw Puzzles

BEST FOR: Practicing visual perception

This activity encourages acute attention to detail while increasing mental speed and short-term memory. Solving a jigsaw puzzle requires spatial-cognitive reasoning on a microscale, whereas navigating through an unfamiliar city with a map uses the same logic on a macroscale.

Individuals with dyslexia often excel in solving puzzles, which invoke their problem-solving brain. But despite having above-average visual-spatial cognitive reasoning abilities, some have an exceedingly tricky time with two-dimensional jigsaw puzzles. When there are many pieces without much diversity, individuals with dyslexia cannot see the trees in the forest.

Start with a 500-piece puzzle with contrasting colors. Or try digital jigsaw puzzles; I find an online puzzle app easier to use than a physical puzzle.

#9. Make a Movie in Your Head

BEST FOR: Visualizing reading comprehension and sustaining attention

This strategy relies on your ability to think in pictures and images. It brings that one step further in asking you to add sequential motion, to make a mental movie. I suggest working on the story comprehension strategy in chapter 4 before attempting this activity.

Pick a short story, article, or chapter in a book that has descriptive language. You can use an audiobook for this if you like. Legendary stories like Robin Hood or fairy tales like Rumpelstiltskin work well for this exercise. Read the story while following these steps:

1. Form a picture of the characters in the story and the scenery where the story takes place. This can be as detailed as you like, in color or black and white.
2. Add to your picture as the story progresses. You may have to alter your images as new information is introduced or settings change.
3. A good stopping point is after a problem has been solved in the story. Pause and try to replay your movie of what you read, without looking at the text.
4. Try reading or listening to the same passage again. Can you add anything to your movie?
5. Consider some more profound questions:

- What can you take away from the passage?
- What details made the passage interesting?
- Was there a moral dilemma? What was it?
- Did you like the outcome of the scene or story? Why or why not?

#10. Soothe Your Eyes

BEST FOR: Mitigating the effects of screen time

During the 2020 COVID quarantine, many of us spent considerably more time in front of a computer screen. Personally, my screen time more than tripled. I found my eyes tired at the end of each day, until someone suggested wearing glasses that block blue light to ease eye strain. I found that this helped. However, research on the benefits of blue light–blocking glasses for eye strain is inconclusive.

Eye strain is not isolated to dyslexia, but because reading and writing take longer, we are likely spending more time in front of our computers than peers in our same line of work. Here are tried-and-true suggested strategies for reducing eye strain when you need to spend time looking at a screen.

- Consult with an optometrist about getting corrective prescription eyeglasses for computer viewing.
- Use lubricating eye drops, sometimes called "artificial tears," to soothe tired eyes. (Avoid drops that promise "red eye relief.")
- Follow the 20-20-20 rule. Every 20 minutes, look up to an object 20 feet away for 20 seconds.
- Work in a well-lit room.
- Explore your screen viewing options, including color filters or overlays, adjustable font size, magnifier, narrator, text-to-voice, and screen contrast.
- Utilize text-to-voice software on your phone or tablet to compose documents while standing or pacing. Use a program linked between devices so you can edit the resulting file on your computer.

Every person is different. Think outside the box; explore your options. Find what works for you.

Conclusion

Individuals with dyslexia, who have strong visual-spatial intelligence, are adept at perceiving and analyzing information in the world around them. Likewise, listening comprehension is typically a strength. Yet both also present challenges, not only to reading and spelling, but to our daily routine. Some of our snafus are even laughable.

In the next chapter we will explore the power and relevance of executive functioning skills: organization, prioritizing, and time management, to name a few.

CHAPTER 6
Master Your Executive Functioning Skills

We use executive functions to manage everyday life. Strong executive functions help us think critically, adapt our behavior, handle our emotions, tolerate stress, and achieve our goals. Dyslexia and difficulties with executive functioning often go hand in hand. The reasons for this aren't always clear. But they could include the impact of a lifetime of being misunderstood, the effects of a coexisting disorder, or the pressure to mask one's faults.

> ### AVERY
> Avery, who uses they/them pronouns, is looking for a new job. Suspecting they were dyslexic, Avery took an online screening test at age 51 and consulted with me about their results. They worked in event planning, developing trade show booths for marketing events that featured the latest technology. Avery has many stories of how their talents aided their previous job, but they're concerned they won't find a similar fit in a new profession. Nonetheless, they want to explore some new career options.
>
> While Avery could recognize their skills at reasoning and making connections, they had not thought much about the role executive functioning had played in their success. But many details had to be considered in planning their projects. Avery could balance all these components and quickly configure a new booth in their mind. They would then send their thoughts to a field designer, who would sketch the drawings. Next a detailer would add the final touches with measurements. Finally, Avery would present the plans to the marketing and sales teams; once approved, they would initiate the project with a team of builders. Avery's executive functioning strengths can be

> described as planning and prioritizing; task initiation; organization; and flexibility. Upon hearing this, Avery laughed and compared themselves to the race-winning tortoise in the famous fable, saying, "I move slow, but I know how to get the job done!"

What Is Executive Function?

Executive function is a blanket term for the set of mental processes that we use to get stuff done. They're the skills that help us plan, attend to, and organize our daily tasks. Most people display both strengths and weaknesses in the skills that make up executive functioning. For instance, someone might have a messy desk but also be very good at planning projects. But for some people, a significant deficit in executive functioning can severely impact their life. Weak executive functioning is most often connected to ADHD. But it can occur with other disorders and learning disabilities, like dyslexia.

What Role Does Executive Functioning Play in the Body/Mind?

Like dyslexia, executive functioning skills are neurological and genetic. We're born with particular aptitudes and preferences wired into our brain. However, many additional factors affect executive functioning strengths and weaknesses. For example, executive functioning is regulated in the brain's frontal lobe; therefore, physical trauma to the forehead can degrade these abilities. Also, one's environment can play a significant role: learned behavior, exposure to toxins, income level, and education attainment all influence the development of executive function. Moreover, executive functioning weaknesses can be a result of learning differences like dyslexia.

Executive functioning is like an office manager. It acts as a filter, keeping out distractions so we can manage daily life and achieve our goals. If our office manager is not good at the job, or not even present, we're flooded with interruptions; as a result, things get out of control and chaotic. Strong executive function helps us control our impulses, focus on our work, make plans, organize, exert self-control, and more. Weak executive functioning can make it hard to make progress toward one's goals, resulting in stress and low self-esteem. Let's take a look at some of the roles that executive function plays in everyday life.

Sustained Attention

There are several types of attention. Sustained attention refers to maintaining the necessary level of mental focus over time, despite distractions, tiredness, or boredom. An example of mental focus might be attending mandatory job training sessions for new software that you don't feel will help you. You're able to listen and remain focused on the presentation even though it doesn't seem relevant to your job. Weak sustained attention might occur when you're trying to read something with complicated wording or sentence structure. No matter how hard you try, you cannot maintain your focus and must read it several times.

The Role of Sustained Attention in Auditory Learning

Listening is an active process. To comprehend what you hear, you must activate your working memory and sustain your attention. This is not easy for people with dyslexia, especially for roughly 30 percent of those who also have ADHD.

Many find it helpful to have a visual aid to accompany verbal instruction. Whether listening to an audio textbook, a college lecturer, or an instructor at a new job, people with ADHD find it hard to simply listen to information. Note-taking apps can make sitting through a lecture a more active experience.

However, people with dyslexia are generally able to attend to audiobooks of interest. Studies show that audiobooks can improve

> motivation and comprehension skills in all readers and help them develop longer periods of sustained attention.

Impulse Control

Also known as inhibition, impulse control is the ability to hold back a behavior by thinking before acting. Most people associate poor impulse control with hyperactive behavior, yet impulse control also involves delayed gratification. You might be tempted by something you want, but if you can't postpone getting it, you might trigger unwanted consequences. For example, you might send an email immediately without checking for clarity because you want to go to lunch, only to find out your message is missing some words.

Working Memory

The executive function of working memory guides and directs our actions. It purposefully keeps us on track, on time, and in control. This is an ongoing, dynamic process. According to psychologist Russell Barkley, our working memory must actively determine incoming information's relevance and alter our plans to get us to our destination, like a GPS. This can be exhausting, especially for those who have weak working memory, a common consequence of dyslexia.

Organization

When we talk about organization in the context of executive function, we mean the ability to create a reliable system that arranges information. Organization is so essential to executive functioning that it's described in three parts: organization of physical objects, time management, and planning/prioritizing. Arranging physical areas like your home and workspace supports work and life efficiency. Being organized is something of a balancing act. Lack of organization can lead to stress. Too much organization can become obsessive-compulsive. We'll address multiple ways that dyslexia impacts the organization of time and space in this chapter.

Time Management

Completing a task or reaching a goal also requires organizing one's time. It's essential we understand how long a task will take, including time for handling unexpected problems. To be effective, one must meet deadlines and understand that time is an essential resource. For someone with dyslexia, it is exceedingly difficult to predict how long language-based tasks, like organizing thoughts into a coherent report or memo, will take. So, someone with dyslexia might over- or undermanage their time. When you lack the ability to manage your time, you can feel as if you're always in a crisis.

Tips and Tricks for Navigating the Workplace

Technology can bridge executive functioning weaknesses in your workplace. Below are some options that are useful for everyone regardless of literacy skills. Many of them are considered common tools for all employees; in other words, they are not accommodations. For suggestions specifically targeting reading and writing support, see chapter 4.

Note-taking apps are becoming second nature for all multitasking jobs. There are numerous applications on the market; many depend on your operating platform but work across devices, including your phone. Several smartpens are available that record while you handwrite notes and create an editable digital file. I suggest trying a few applications to see what works best for your needs.

Organizing apps offer support for executive functioning by helping you keep a schedule. Online calendars sync to applications that help you prioritize. Project applications assist you in breaking down projects into manageable tasks to meet a due date and tracking progress. There are several self-check apps available to help regulate sustained attention and inhibit impulsive behaviors.

> The technology is endless and changing exponentially, so explore the possibilities. Besides, it is my experience that employers are more open to applications that support executive functioning skills than ones that support a learning disability.

Planning/Prioritizing

As a separate executive functioning skill, planning/prioritizing is the ability to look ahead and determine what is needed and in what order to accomplish a task. To succeed, you must break down larger projects (the big picture) into manageable tasks (the details), then decide where to put your attention and effort first. Working with details isn't easy for people with dyslexia, so we'll discuss this further in this chapter.

Task Initiation

Task initiation is the mental effort of beginning a task. One might have a problem starting any size project regardless of motivation. While this might simply be called procrastination, we need to look for a deeper reason why. Several things might keep one from starting a task, including fear of failure, low self-esteem, and not having the tools one needs. When one cannot begin tasks, responsibilities add up, creating a continual sense of feeling behind.

Cognitive Flexibility

Cognitive flexibility is the mental ability to shift one's focus and revise a plan when faced with obstacles. Someone who has difficulty with cognitive flexibility does not adapt to change; they continue the same behavior despite complications. Seeking out new experiences and creative thinking can encourage cognitive flexibility. In addition, practicing mental flexibility leads to increased brain functioning and lower stress levels. This is typically a strength for individuals with dyslexia, who tend to be creative problem solvers. In fact, it's an ability that enables many people with dyslexia to find work-arounds to their literacy challenges.

Emotional Control

Emotional control is the ability to manage our feelings in order to complete tasks. It's the ability to stay calm and bounce back from disruptive emotions, without deeper feelings of discouragement or shame settling in. People with weak emotional control experience quick changes in their feelings; friends or colleagues might describe them as a loose cannon. However, a person with dyslexia may feel self-conscious and internalize their emotions, only seeming to be in control. Either way, a person struggling to keep their emotions in check will likely feel drained and find it challenging to achieve their goals.

What Are the Executive Functioning Challenges for a Dyslexic Individual?

The relationship between dyslexia and executive functioning can be a bit counterintuitive. It's important to note that dyslexia does not directly cause executive functioning problems. Not all individuals with dyslexia will have weak executive functioning; in fact, some individuals with dyslexia have strong executive functioning skills. But others will find aspects of executive functioning challenging. In some cases, executive functioning issues are affected by coexisting conditions like ADHD.

Stress and anxiety are familiar to someone with dyslexia. Not surprisingly, executive functions can be impaired by the high levels of stress and anxiety that dyslexia might bring to the table. Additionally, low levels of self-esteem and self-confidence impede one's ability to predict and accept success.

Interestingly, executive skills' effectiveness can differ from work to home. Psychologists Peg Dawson and Richard Guare report that executive strengths at work shift to weaknesses at home 65 percent of the time. For example, you might be skilled at time management at work, never being late to a meeting. Still, you are constantly late picking your kids up at their afterschool activities.

Starting and Managing Tasks

Let's examine what challenges a person with dyslexia might face when beginning and overseeing a task.

Task initiation: The mental effort to begin a task can be hindered by fear of failure, low self-esteem, or lack of support.

Planning/prioritizing: This requires breaking down big ideas into details, but people with dyslexia tend to see the forest, not the trees.

Time management: Predicting how much time is needed depends on one's ability to organize their thoughts.

Organization: Preparing a physical space and gathering materials needed can involve attention to detail that's lacking with dyslexia.

Focus

It's easier to sustain our attention when it feels like we can grasp the ideas being presented. But at times, some information or tasks will simply be beyond our reach because of poor working memory, low literacy levels, or the presentation of the material. For example, your partner rattles off a sequence of items to remember to do when you come home, but it sounds like a random list that you can't make sense of. Or your boss presents a new marketing tactic with no visual elements to illustrate the concept. You try to focus, but you're unable to attend to rote, verbal information.

Organization of Time

Everything about time seems to be a challenge for someone with dyslexia. For example, imagine reading an analog clock when you can't determine the orientation of the hand. Or trying to decode Roman numerals. So, logically, organizing time is problematic. The dyslexic person's tendency for global creative thinking makes it difficult to pay attention to details when organizing a schedule. Managing a monthly or seasonal calendar might take several rechecks. You might have to reschedule multiple appointments because you forgot to build in prep and transition time. Some details might be overlooked, or you might connect an event to the wrong day, date, or time.

Working Memory

Remember, working memory integrates information in a short time. So for executive function, your working memory must:

Attend to information being presented.

Break apart the incoming information or word and quickly determine how to respond.

Effective working memory means we must determine the trees of the forest. We cannot simply utilize the vague, bigger picture.

Feeling Overwhelmed

A person feels overwhelmed when emotions catch them off guard or have built up unnoticed. An individual with dyslexia might find themselves in a position in which a literacy activity has taken longer than expected. A shift in job responsibilities may mean they need to find additional support. A change in schedule means they have less time to read important documents. These kinds of situations can trigger embarrassment or fear of being found out. Overwhelming emotions can lead to low self-confidence and self-doubt about one's qualifications.

Stress Tolerance

Dealing with stress engages many executive functions and highly impacts our wellness. Stress tolerance means being able to manage obstacles or uncertainties and turn them around for positive or negative results. Good stress tolerance encourages motivation, which develops greater focus. Low stress tolerance brings frustration, which can lead to sadness and anxiety, even helplessness.

Choosing the Right Career

> A survey of 71 successful adults with dyslexia found that those who felt successful reported that their executive functioning skills were highly regarded in their job and that they were provided with support from colleagues and technology.
>
> To help you focus on a career that will match your executive function skills, I recommend taking a survey to understand your strengths and weaknesses. I list some options in the Resources.
>
> Some dyslexia-friendly career paths include landscape or interior designer, architect, inventor, engineer, builder, scientist, lawyer, therapist, researcher, teacher, handyman, plumber, electrician, actor, author, historian, event planner, and human resource specialist.
>
> I suggest leaning into your executive functioning strengths, while working to improve one weakness at a time. Strategies at the end of this chapter will help.

The Key Is to Know Yourself

Metacognition is the ability to be aware of your awareness: to know yourself and how you think. A recent UK study reports that adults with dyslexia who are strong at goal setting and understanding their own thinking process are happier in their jobs and possess positive self-worth. People with self-awareness feel a sense of efficacy and internal control that provides confidence and satisfaction.

Consider this scenario: Bryan, serving in the military, was in an intense academic training program in his field of expertise. He wanted to do well. While his peers spent every waking moment drilling the material, Bryan knew he could not use rote memorization to learn. Instead, based on prior experience, he understood how he learned best. Bryan had to comprehend the concepts by studying how they were interconnected. Also, to internalize the lessons, Bryan had to study while being active; for example, he'd often shoot baskets during his breaks while drilling himself on the material. Thanks to his self-awareness, Bryan not only passed the course, he also graduated top of his class.

Be Honest about Your Strengths and Weaknesses

Sometimes it is easier to avoid facing our weaknesses in executive functioning. We dodge the pile of paperwork or avoid preplanning a hectic day. However, avoidance only creates the elephant in the room; tasks don't just go away because we pretend not to see them. By not tackling a difficult challenge, you are likely denying yourself the ability to thrive. Facing our challenges allows us to embrace our strengths.

Strategies to Improve Your Executive Functioning

This chapter's strategies are focused on improving your executive functioning skills. I suggest focusing on improving one skill at a time until you feel a difference. Remember that you may have to revisit a learned skill from time to time. Many of these strategies center on organization and planning, which is particularly relevant to individuals with dyslexia. But not everyone has the same weaknesses. For broader help with executive functioning, refer to the Resources.

#1. Do a Workplace Check-In

BEST FOR: Organizing your functional workspace

This strategy sets you up to organize a supportive workspace, by checking in on both your environment and your temperament. Answer the prompts and consider making the relevant changes to your work area.

1. Does your workspace include everything you need to do your job? Are all tools and materials accessible? Does anything need to be replenished?
2. Is your workspace free from clutter? What's the best time of day to reorganize and declutter?

3. Do you have a supportive chair, a stand-up desk, or ergonomically appropriate gear? Consider your posture and physique while you work. What would help protect your body from injury or strain?

4. What's the auditory environment like? Do you need music or sound-filtering headphones to lessen distraction and aid your focus?

Reevaluate your workspace from time to time. Ask yourself: What's working for me? What needs to change? What factors affect my comfort and productivity? Make changes appropriately.

#2. Be the Master of Your Schedule

BEST FOR: Organizing your time by creating a daily routine for better productivity

Individuals with dyslexia often need to work harder than their peers to accomplish the same task, especially reading and writing. That means you need to become a master at organizing your time so you can get everything done. Use these prompts to plan the most productive schedule possible.

1. What's your most efficient time of day, when your mind is sharpest and you're best able to focus on your work? Plan your routine so this time period is protected from distractions and mundane tasks. Pre-pack your lunch or bring coffee with you, for example, so you don't have to leave your desk while you're at your most productive.

2. How long can you work before needing a break? Does that change over the course of the day? Spend a week tracking when your attention wanes, and schedule small breaks accordingly. Include longer intervals for lunch, taking a walk, or other away-from-the-desk activities. Use an alarm on your phone or device to remind you when it's time to take breaks.

3. Do you get distracted by your phone or by emails? Try checking messages only at specific times, and otherwise not accessing them.

Studies have indicated that bundling responses to emails and texts can save time in a day.

As with your workspace, evaluate your scheduling situation from time to time. Ask what's working and what needs to change.

#3. Evaluate Your Time

BEST FOR: Managing tasks

To prevent being overwhelmed, or putting something off, it helps to be able to **accurately** estimate the time that routine responsibilities take—the key word being accurately. To develop that skill, this exercise (with details borrowed from Dawson and Guare's The Smart but Scattered Guide to Success) prompts you to compare your estimates with reality. Here's how it works:

1. Create a table with five columns. You can do this on paper or with digital tools, however you prefer. But it should be in a format you can access while you're working.
2. Label the columns from left to right: Activity, Estimated Time, Start, Stop, Actual Time.
3. List your daily activities in the Activity column: "Check emails," "Update database," "Restock inventory," etc.
4. Draw a line under each activity to create a row across all columns.
5. In column two, write down your best estimate for how much time each activity typically takes you.
6. Keep your document with you as you go through your day. As you begin each listed task, write down the time when you start. Upon completion, write down your stopping time.
7. At the end of the day, complete column five with actual times and see how they compare to your estimates.

Repeat this exercise over the course of a few weeks. See how close you can bring your estimates to reality. Also take note of which times of day you are most productive. Try shifting tasks to different start times. You might be surprised by the outcome.

#4. Mind Mapping

> **BEST FOR:** Ordering and sequencing a plan to complex problems or schedules

With this strategy, you'll create a visual representation of your schedule, helping you see the work that's ahead of you and make decisions accordingly.

You will need one or more of these sets of items, depending on your preference:

- A whiteboard and fine-tip dry-erase markers
- Blank white paper and fine-tip markers
- Sticky notes and a board or surface to organize them on

For this mind map, you will brainstorm all that you have to do during a specific period of time—a busy day, a week, whatever interval you choose. Represent that in the center of your writing area by writing "My day," "Week of March 3," or whatever designation is appropriate.

Next, add branches representing each event or task you must attend to. If you like, you can create separate branches representing each day, and branch that day's agenda off of it.

Draw lines off of each branch to list the details: time, place, agenda, materials, and whatever else will help your planning.

Individuals with dyslexia think in big pictures. A mind map helps you begin with the big picture and list details at different levels. Use your map to guide yourself as you work through the time period you've mapped. Look for conflicts: Are some events scheduled too close together or too far apart? Do you have the resources to complete each task? Would it help to shift anything to a different day or time?

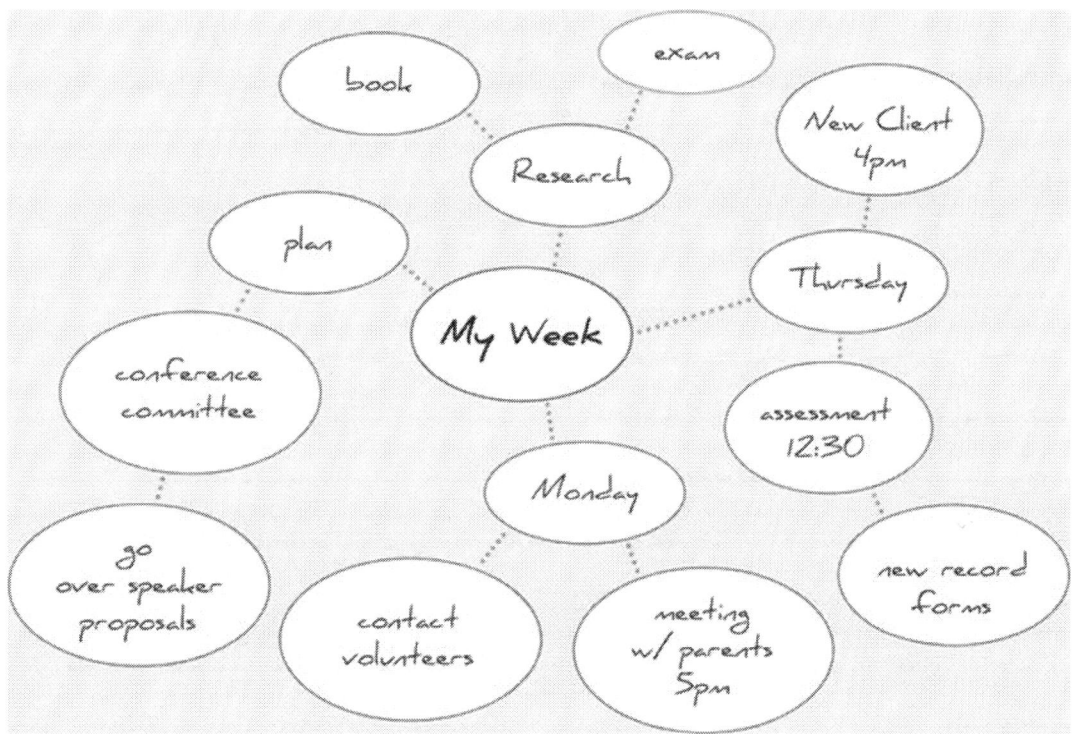

#5. Preparing and Transitions

BEST FOR: Time management

Time management does not stop at fixing tasks into a schedule. It also takes time to prepare and to move from one task to another. We need to be certain we have all the materials and resources needed to begin. We may need to factor in driving time or other transportation, setting up, and reorganizing a workspace afterward.

To do this, Dawson and Guare recommend applying these steps to your schedule, calendar, or mind map:

1. List all the critical elements to carry out your plan, including materials, personnel, time, workspace, and data.
2. Ask yourself what essential tools you will need. What do you already have? What will you need to purchase or rent?

3. Identify the skill sets you will need. Do you possess the needed expertise? Will you have to learn something new or bring in someone else? What obstacles might you encounter in doing so?

4. Break down each step in performing your task and write them in order. Estimate how long each step will take and attach a deadline to each.

5. Consider who else might need to be involved, how they will help, and when they'll be needed.

6. Lastly, review your plan in light of the above details and modify what will not work.

This information can be written as notes on a calendar or mind map.

#6. Tackle Household Chores

BEST FOR: Task initiation

Household chores can pile up after a long week at work. They seem overwhelming but avoiding them will cause more stress.

In The Smart but Scattered Guide to Success, Peg Dawson recommends making two lists of household chores: low-effort chores (things you do easily) and high-effort chores (things you struggle with). Then evaluate the list with these questions:

1. Look for common themes. Which executive functioning skills are called upon for your easy list? Which are on your hard list? The result might reveal your at-home executive functioning strengths and weaknesses. You might excel at keeping a neat desktop in your office but dread straightening up the kitchen counter.

2. Consider other factors that influence your attitude toward these tasks: Are some of the chores on your hard list physically exerting? If so, in what way?

3. If you have a partner, have them fill out a similar list and compare notes. Maybe you have complementary outlooks. For example, washing windows might be on your high-effort list but no big deal for your partner.
4. Divvy up the high-effort chores or consider hiring someone for them. Group low-effort chores together and plan to knock out a bunch of them when you can.

Be realistic; you do not need to tackle everything each week. Prioritize tasks that cause you stress when they are not completed. Develop a coping strategy for achieving them, like listening to an audiobook or a favorite podcast, or taking frequent breaks.

#7. Checking Your Work

BEST FOR: Self-monitoring

Are there certain tasks you like to rush through? For example, you might have a habit of writing emails and sending them without reviewing them first. My family used to tease me about my texts, which often did not make sense until I extended a grammar and spelling app to my phone. Sometimes it's easier to avoid our mistakes, to try sweeping them under the rug, so to speak, than to face them.

For this exercise, identify the tasks or situations that you rush through. These might be responsibilities you wish you could avoid or ones you've been criticized or teased about. Then apply these steps to each situation:

1. What supports might help you avoid errors? For example, grammar and spellcheckers or a reading application. Consider creating a checklist or cue to follow, which will remind you to look at details before considering the task complete.
2. For communication tasks, put yourself in the receiver's shoes before you send anything. Will this make sense to them?

3. Ask yourself guided questions to make sure your information is correct. For example: What's the exact time of an event? What will I need to bring? How much time will this take? What are the costs involved?

Not everything you do can be monitored. But by building a habit of checking your work whenever possible, you lessen opportunities for a sense of dread or embarrassment.

#8. Helping You Remember

BEST FOR: Compensate for your working memory

Studies have shown that our working memory can only hold between one and four things at a time. But we can compensate or accommodate for our working memory's limits.

Keep lists. I have recently started using a phone app so my lists are accessible anywhere. I kept forgetting my handwritten lists at home.

Put things where you can see them. If you need to remember to bring something with you to work or on a trip, put it by the door. If you worry you'll step over it, put it on your car's driver seat or attach a bright note to the steering wheel.

Follow routines. A routine is an automatic action that relies on subconscious or long-term memory, no decision-making needed. Maybe you have a standard batch of items you buy at the grocery store once a week. Perhaps each morning you empty the dishwasher. We don't need to remember the things that we do every day; we just do them.

Use technology. Supportive resources like planning software, cloud-based document archives, automated bill payment, and find-my-phone apps can lighten the load of what we need to remember.

Surround yourself with encouragement. Studies show that motivation and attention aid better working memory outcomes. Keep up your relationships with friends and family who you can count on for emotional support. Post favorite inspirational quotes and aphorisms where you'll see them regularly.

#9. Reframe Anxious Feelings

BEST FOR: Feeling overwhelmed

When overwhelming feelings wash over us, we cannot think rationally. Intense feelings impede our ability to engage in daily tasks. Unexpected changes to a routine can cause feelings of fear and anxiety.

Individuals with dyslexia may experience temporary bouts of overwhelming feelings, usually brought on from a sense of not being in control of their time, especially when there is a deadline pending for work or school. In some cases, overwhelming feelings can cause a panic attack or paralyzed feeling. Or one might lash out at friends and family trying to help.

Here are some options for staying on track when feeling overwhelmed:

Accept the anxious feelings. You can feel anxious and still complete your tasks.

Reframe damaging thoughts. Don't make a tough time into a referendum on who you are.

Just breathe. Try your favorite meditation techniques or the breathing exercise in chapter 2.

Step away from the situation. Go for a walk, step into the hall, take a coffee break.

Use your resources. Ask for help from colleagues. Work with your calendar or planner to create a new and more realistic schedule. Do research to see how other people have handled this problem.

Remind yourself with healthy self-talk: "I have been here before. It always gets better."

Meditation, music, exercise, self-talk, and other relaxation tactics, even for a short time, can help calm and refocus your emotions. It can also help to just get started on the task at hand. In most cases, overwhelming feelings subside as control of the situation returns.

#10. Microproductivity

BEST FOR: Breaking apart a large job into smaller parts

Large tasks might appear unmanageable or unapproachable. Microproductivity is a buzzword for the segmentation of more significant projects into doable parts. To decompose a project:

1. Define the project parameters. When is it due? How will completeness be determined? What are the limitations for resources, time, personnel, etc.?
2. Use a top-down approach to break the project into segments of relatively equal length in time or scope, divided by logical milestones. For example, if you're writing a large report, you might allow one week for researching and gathering materials, another week to complete a first draft, a third to review and revise, and a fourth week for final proofing, printing, and delivery of the copies.
3. Subdivide each segment further as needed. In the example, you might spend the first two days of week one pulling information from an archive, one day interviewing relevant sources, and two days winnowing the information to its essentials and creating an outline.
4. Arrange the steps so they fit with your work preferences. How long can you or your team members stay focused or remain productive? Perhaps a whole day of archival research is too taxing, and it would be better to break up that time with interviews and outlining.

5. Be sure your schedule includes breaks, with time for stretching, walks, or other physical movement. Respect your well-being when planning.

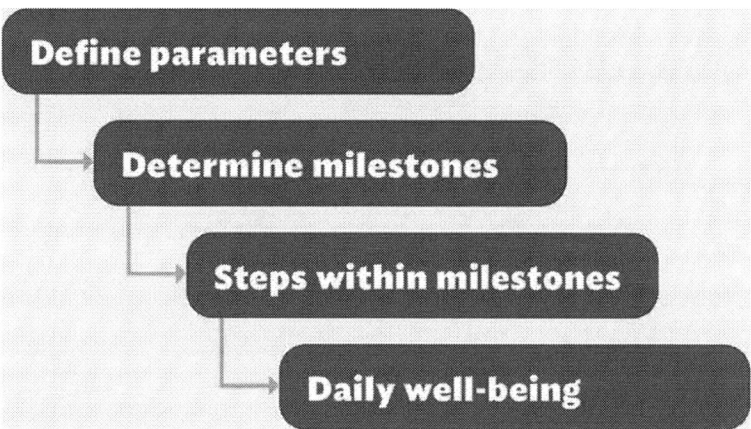

Conclusion

Like so many other aspects of dyslexia, its relationship with executive functions produces a combination of strengths and weaknesses. However, we can improve our particular executive functioning by considering how we plan, organize, and attend to tasks. Concerning dyslexia, some weaknesses in executive functioning are predictable and therefore manageable with practice. Still, we will all have our own strengths and struggles. Think of your executive functions as tools that you can learn to use better over time.

CHAPTER 7

Embrace Your Strengths

When told dyslexia was a gift, one young scholar reportedly answered, "Where can I return it?" But as we've been saying since chapter 1, dyslexia really does bring strengths and advantages as well as challenges and obstacles. In this chapter we will take a deeper look at what these gifts are and how to use the strengths of dyslexia to your advantage. By embracing dyslexia, you can become the best you.

> ### SHEELA
>
> Sheela first realized that her reading and writing struggles were due to dyslexia when her two sons were diagnosed. She'd never considered her struggles unique; Sheela thought everyone worked as hard as she did. Growing up, no one ever made her feel different. In fact, she was a straight-A student through elementary school. But when her first son was diagnosed, Sheela learned that dyslexia was inherited, and for the first time she had a name for her literacy tribulations.
>
> As an adult, Sheela reports being a slow reader. Writing anything can take several hours to days, even if it's a simple email; she must edit and rewrite it several times. Sheela doesn't read out loud, except to her youngest son. Even with children's books, she will stammer.
>
> Nevertheless, Sheela shares that living with dyslexia has not diminished her confidence. In fact, her confidence has helped her overcome her struggles. At an early age, she discovered a passion for dance and performance and developed a can-do-anything mindset that carried her through a master's degree in child life. Today, Sheela uses her talents to empathize with others' pain in her work as a child life specialist supporting kids coping with illness, trauma, and loss.

> Sheela feels fortunate to be working in a career that she's passionate about. She credits much of her success to her parents' encouragement and her grad school professors who supported her. She recognizes a deep drive to make others happy, which she credits to her interconnected reasoning skills, a common strength that comes with dyslexia.

The Left-Brain and Right-Brain Relationship in a Dyslexic Individual

You might be familiar with the notion that the right side of the human brain is connected to creativity, while the left side is involved in logic. Though that's a simplification, the gist is that the right brain is associated with big-picture thinking. Broad ideas are formed in our creative mind, relationships are connected, and inferences shape profound conclusions. But these cognitive processes are slower and allow more questions to arise.

In contrast, the left brain is associated with more precise thinking; it's detail-oriented, forming quick, decisive conclusions. Through scientific research, we know that the left side of the brain is also responsible for many language details, like producing individual sounds and syntax. However, most people with dyslexia rely heavily on their right brain to read.

Individuals with dyslexia think differently. The specializations in the brain's physical structures have led scientists to believe that there is a trade-off between precise, rapid processing and producing broader concepts. One cannot be gifted in one area without a compromise from the other.

There Are Many Inherent Strengths That Come with Dyslexia

A person with dyslexia most likely will have varied, interacting strengths in performing visual-spatial tasks, making connections, and predicting patterns, to name a few. These strengths can overlap. For instance, someone's ability to predict patterns might help them connect data points that seem unrelated. Likewise, a single strength can bring about many outcomes; for example, empathy can generate multiple perspectives to a solution, emotion, or cause. There is no doubt that our inherent strengths are the root of many aptitudes.

Sometimes we lack the confidence to believe in our skills. But no matter how reluctant we may be to believe in ourselves, we each have a small voice somewhere deep inside that whispers, "You've got this."

So let's turn away from the challenges of dyslexia and take a closer look at the gifts dyslexia can bring.

Problem-Solving

Forest rangers watch for fires from a tower that lets them view the whole forest, not by staring at a single tree. People with dyslexia are quick to recognize a problem because it is a big idea, and big ideas are our specialty. The dyslexic brain uses a top-down approach to solving problems, starting with identifying the problem itself. After collecting the gist, the dyslexic brain works to connect details, formulating a solution. Problem-solving is useful for careers like project manager, engineer, designer, air traffic controller, stay-at-home parent, and much more. In fact, it's hard to imagine a profession that doesn't need problem solvers.

Seeing a Topic from All Angles

Individuals with dyslexia often use an interdisciplinary, or broad, approach to solving problems. They consider all angles to a problem. Trying various approaches, they often borrow and adapt from other sources. Because of this, a person who has dyslexia often falls into becoming a "Jack of all trades," knowledgeable in many professions instead of highly specialized in one area. This wide knowledge base can lead to creative approaches that others had not imagined.

Creativity

Creativity is the act of bringing a new idea into being, whether it's an abstract concept or a physical expression, like a painting, musical performance, or manufactured product. The dyslexic brain likes to connect relationships, explore new ideas, and consider subjects from different angles, all of which support creative thinking. Creativity is a component of almost every human endeavor: art, business, medicine, storytelling, comedy, design; even scientific research benefits from creativity. In just about everything we do and every decision we make, there's room for a creative touch.

Vision

Individuals with dyslexia are goal setters. Typically, they are persistent in reaching the goals they set. Determined to do well, they do not let distractions get in their way. One study found that almost 35 percent of entrepreneurs in America have dyslexia. Among the reasons for their success was a clear and persistent vision of their goal. In addition, these individuals could communicate their clear idea to others, who could join their cause.

Intuition

In researching famous people with dyslexia, I found that "intuition" kept popping out. Many reported that they just knew how to do something. They did not always use tangible evidence when making decisions but trusted their gut. For instance, one young comedian told of being able to walk into a room and capture the vibe of the crowd. They were able to read the room, summing up the mood and demographics within minutes. While performing, they were able to gauge when to finish. When asked how they knew all this, they responded, "Doesn't everybody?"

Famous Dyslexic Inventors throughout History

> Consider these celebrated inventors and scientists who are believed to have had dyslexia. They brought us innovative ideas despite a clear struggle to read and write—and perhaps because of the gifts that came with those struggles.
>
> Alexander Graham Bell (1847–1922)
>
> Jacques Dubochet (1942–present): Swiss biochemist and Nobel Prize winner in chemistry
>
> Thomas Edison (1847–1931)
>
> Henry Ford (1863–1947)
>
> Galileo Galilei (1564–1642): Italian astronomer, physicist, and engineer
>
> William P. Lear (1902–1978): First mass manufacturer of business jet aircraft in the world
>
> Nikola Tesla (1856–1943): Invented the modern alternating current electricity supply system
>
> Eli Whitney (1765–1825): Inventor of the cotton gin
>
> The Wright brothers: Made their first successful flight on December 17, 1903
>
> Unfortunately, less is known about dyslexia among inventors in previous eras who were women or belonged to diverse racial and ethnic groups. If they struggled in school, they may have had to drop out to join the workforce. It is also possible that their successes were not recorded or were credited to white men.

Resilience

Resilience is the ability to bounce back from adversity. For most of us, dyslexia has made life more difficult. As children, many of us had to face obstacles every day we went to school. As adults, we have the freedom to accept paths of less resistance. But knowing what it's like to persevere through adversity, we may choose to follow a challenging road to achieve our goals. Many times we work harder than our peers on similar tasks; we tend to keep that struggle to ourselves because we're willing to do what it takes. When dyslexia knocks us down, we've learned to pick ourselves up and move forward.

Determination

In her book Grit, Angela Lee Duckworth identifies passion and perseverance as attributes of those who succeed. Duckworth observed that talent has little to do with success. Goal-minded individuals, willing to fail and try again, were more likely to achieve success than their fixed-mindset peers. In most cases, those of us who live with dyslexia find things challenging but not impossible.

Empathy and Character

A recent study (2020) found that children with dyslexia have greater emotional capacity to understand others' feelings. Although this study was on children, in my experience, the same is true for dyslexics of any age. People with dyslexia are more aware of emotions in themselves and in others. And this empathy is the root of many interpersonal character strengths. A 2018 survey of adults in the United States and United Kingdom reported that fairness, kindness, and good judgment were among the hallmark character strengths in adults with dyslexia.

Considering Others' Perspectives

Individuals with dyslexia find it easy to consider other perspectives when solving problems. Debate isn't typically their strength; they instinctively see both sides of an issue. In my practice, the most common request for adult evaluations occurs from students in law school. There are not many famous dyslexic lawyers. My theory is that while individuals with dyslexia are gifted in analytical skills that are important to law, they are not the ones in court arguing a case. If you have dyslexia, you might have too much empathy for the other's point of view and prefer to work behind the scenes.

You Can Use These Skills to Your Advantage

Knowing yourself is half the journey in life; to succeed, you must sell yourself, too. Undeniably, having dyslexia has not been easy. But you can reframe your struggles and highlight your talents. For example, lean on your strength of connectiveness to bring a stellar team around you to cover the gaps in your abilities. Or envision a design that you bring to the best drafter or artists to render it and complete the details. Maybe you are a gifted storyteller and can use voice-to-text to get your words on paper.

Society Is Slowly Embracing Neurodiversity

Have you seen the TV show The Big Bang Theory? It's just one of many television shows and movies that highlight out-of-the-box thinkers and people whose brains function differently.

Neurodiversity is the concept that people whose brains function differently are part of the normal variation in the human population. Coined in 1998 by Judy Singer, it promotes the view that people with so-called disabilities like autism can be recognized for the strengths that their condition enables, while not underestimating the struggles. Neurodiverse minds, including people with autism, ADHD, dyslexia, bipolar, and other conditions, are credited with bringing about much of the innovative technology we value today.

Workplaces and Schools Are Becoming More Accommodating

Along with recognizing your strengths, it's important to remember that the challenges of dyslexia are becoming less and less burdensome. There's a growing trend to make accommodations accessible to all. For example, voice-to-text and digital books would have been tagged accommodations in the past; today, both are easily accessible. There are even voice-to-text apps with vocabulary for specific careers, like law or medicine. In the past, technical accommodations of this sort were unaffordable or inaccessible for personal use.

In college, professors' notes are published before, and available during and after, a lecture. Modern note-taking apps allow for the lecturer's notes to be downloaded and interacted with during classes. Study groups to enable students to grapple with course material are common, and most colleges offer free subject tutoring for all students.

Efficiency is valued in the modern workplace. Many workplaces allow personnel to use their own personal devices to access multiple technical platforms. Many platforms have embedded accessible features to accommodate reading, written communication, and language challenges. PowerPoint and other presentation platforms allow creative thinkers to organize their thoughts using a visual-auditory format.

Find a Career Where You'll Thrive

You might be under the assumption that you need an advanced degree to snag the job of your dreams. Not true. There are jobs at all levels that require high-order thinking skills. In one study, adults with dyslexia placed personal accomplishments higher in measuring job success than their peers. In other words, they found a sense of fulfillment in careers that used their abilities to accomplish their goals. You do not always need an advanced degree to utilize your cognitive strengths.

Below are a few of many routes to finding your niche:

Work with a career coach. These individuals are trained and skilled in matching personality profiles to job types. Some of them also help with resumes and job searches.

Take a career/personality test. These questionnaires (see Resources) are helpful to expose strengths useful in the job market.

> Get help from resume writing centers. The staff is trained to help you highlight your talents and experiences and format your resume to best catch the notice of hiring managers.
>
> Join LinkedIn or other career networks to collaborate and communicate with people in your desired field.

Building Up Your Strengths Will Help Boost Your Confidence

Cognitive behavioral psychology tells us knowing our strengths and accepting our weaknesses will boost our self-confidence. So, identifying your strengths is important. But I've had clients get stuck here, worried because they cannot identify any gifted areas. When we speak of strengths, we're talking about the unique way your mind works, not outward talents or high achievements.

Celebrate what you are good at; do not overthink it. Focus on the unique way your brain works, using the strengths outlined in this chapter as a starting point. Consider the solutions and work-arounds you've had to develop in your life to compensate for your dyslexia and achieve your goals. As you acknowledge your inherent strengths, apply them to everyday opportunities. Remember, completing milestones of any size brings about a feeling of success, building confidence to tackle the next goal. Whoopi Goldberg testifies: "I am where I am because I believe in all possibilities."

Strategies to Build Your Strengths

Let's review the strengths we've touched on in this chapter: big picture thinking, creativity, connectiveness, predicting patterns, problem-solving, understanding multiple perspectives, storytelling, intuition, and goal setting. We've also discussed attributes such as empathy, resilience, determination, and confidence.

The following strategies are meant to help you explore the potential of those overlapping talents. You might sharpen underused strengths or make the most of ones you are already using. Be sure to consider how you might use certain skills at home but have not thought to bring the same talent to your workplace or vice versa. For example, a person skilled in storytelling might try to tell stories in their job; doing so could help them connect with clients or explain procedures to staff. Or an innovator at work may not realize they can plan a vacation or design the landscape for their backyard with the same creative thinking. Try crossing over some of your strengths between the domains of your life.

#1. What Are Your Talents?

BEST FOR: Identifying your workplace strengths

This activity will ask you to informally evaluate your strengths in your workplace. Also consider the strengths test listed in Resources.

1. Use these prompts to brainstorm what works for you and what does not:

   - What do you find easy to accomplish at work? What's your first go-to when you have a choice of tasks? What do you enjoy best?
   - What areas of your work are more challenging? What are the tasks that you tend to put off or that take a lot of time?
   - What skills of yours do others tend to point out or commend you for? What compliments have you received?
   - What workplace milestones have you accomplished in the past? What skills helped you achieve those goals?

2. Decide where to take things next.

   Take note of your strengths: Can they be fostered to better serve your team or job?

   Evaluate more challenging tasks: Can you delegate or swap those out to your team members? Or schedule them for times when they'll be easier to work on?

Be realistic about what changes you can accomplish. And consider the time frame they will take.

3. Consider seeking a mentor to share your goals with.

#2. Building Relationships

BEST FOR: Collaborating with colleagues who may have the same or opposing strengths

This strategy will help you determine how your strengths fit into your team or work environment and how to consider other people's profiles when working together.

As in any relationship, all players matter; each comes to the job with their own profile of strengths and weaknesses. When we relate to each other, each of us does so through our own perspective. Same or opposing strengths in a team can conflict or complement each other.

Are there strengths of your team members or coworkers that counteract your weaknesses? For instance, you're good at working with customers; your coworker is meticulous about entering data. This could be a positive relationship.

Are there opposing strengths and weaknesses in your team? For example, your strength is time management, and your coworker is late to every meeting. This most likely is frustrating. To handle it remember to:

- Try to understand their perspective.
- Look for the strengths they bring to the job.
- Be sensitive to how you might also frustrate them.
- If you are comfortable, have a conversation identifying the conflicting strength/weakness and what can be done about it.
- If necessary, decide on boundaries that will make the situation tolerable. Or bring in a supervisor to resolve the conflict. But being

aware of such conflicts is usually enough to lessen the issue. In most cases, we can agree to be different.

#3. Keep a Routine

BEST FOR: Adding structure for a creative persona

Planning some structure into your day can allow you to get tasks done and be flexible in the in-between times, promoting your creative brainpower.

Creative people like flexibility and freedom. But too much freedom in their day can result in chores piling up. To prevent this, one of my clients suggests following a schedule, saying, "Keeping a routine saves me from thinking about all the things I should be doing. I have more flexibility to do the things I want to do, that make me feel good." Here's how it works:

Wake up generally at the same time of day and do things in the same order: the uninteresting but important stuff first, like checking email, paying bills, and making the bed.

Chunk your routine around pivotal points in your day, like grocery shopping, household chores, mandatory meetings, or walking the dog. In between fixed daily tasks, you have the flexible time to use as you choose.

#4. Time to Think

BEST FOR: Drawing out communication from innovative thinkers

When you are lost in your thoughts, your coworkers or life partners may not know what you are thinking. You may appear distracted, self-engrossed, and unresponsive to others' ideas.

Most of our inventors were known to be dreamers. Many were penalized at school for not paying attention to the lessons. What often looks like daydreaming is inventive thinking, which can be misinterpreted. To better communicate your intentions during those times, try these tactics:

Be aware of yourself in space.

Compartmentalize your time. Leave time in your schedule for your mind to wander so you won't be as tempted otherwise.

Be present when you're with others. Respond to what they're saying so they know you're paying attention.

When a new idea pops into your mind, capture it with an app or jot it down for later.

Have a dedicated space and time to work and a signal that lets others know you can't be disturbed so you won't have to worry about your thinking time being interrupted.

Communicate your thoughts and ideas with those close to you so they'll realize what you can contribute.

Place value on others' input; take time to listen to their ideas as well as sharing your own.

#5. Deploying Empathy

BEST FOR: Fostering connection

This exercise will ask you to explore your empathy and use it to build relationships and understanding in your workplace.

Individuals with dyslexia are often gifted at grasping relationships. They know what it is like to be the underdog, work hard, and face obstacles. A recent study reports that empathy in the workplace has slowed down. Yet 82 percent of CEOs realize the value of having an empathetic work environment.

As a person with dyslexia, you can bring much-needed empathy to your place of work. Writing for Psychology Today, executive coach Marcia Reynolds tells us that to increase our empathy, we must follow these practices:

1. Be quiet, inside and out. Meditation, taking a walk, and other calming activities can quiet our brains.
2. Fully watch as well as listen. Engross yourself in others' stories. Watch and listen; don't speak.
3. Ask yourself what you are feeling. What is your emotional reaction to what other people tell you or how they behave?
4. Test your instinct. Communicate your emotions to others. You might gauge what they're feeling through their body language or words.

Like anything else, practice makes perfect. If empathy comes easily to you, you might be a model to others.

#6. Storytelling in the Workplace

BEST FOR: Persuasive communication through storytelling

This strategy will guide you in the use of storytelling to connect with people, share a vision, or give a meaningful message in your workplace.

Who doesn't like a good story? Storytelling is gaining popularity as a highly effective tool in the workplace. Stories are engaging; they create a movie in the listener's mind. Leaders are using stories to motivate employees, create cultural identity, and empower employees. Storytelling involves relating past episodes to understand current or future events. While anyone can tell a story, storytelling is a recognized gift for some with dyslexia.

While you can use any structural model for storytelling, I suggest you begin with the seven-step story spine model. This was created by Kenn Adams, author of The Art of Spontaneous Theater:

1. Once upon a time . . .
2. Everyday . . .
3. But, one day . . .
4. Because of that . . .

5. Because of that . . . (repeat as many times as needed)

6. Until finally . . .

7. And ever since then . . .

For example, let's apply this to create an advertising campaign for a fictitious app called Locker:

Last week, my dog ate my homework.
This has been an ongoing problem.
But I found a solution. I now keep my homework safe in organized files on Locker.
That way, I can always access what I need and turn in my assignments with one click.
And my dog can stick to his kibble.
Of course, you can use Locker, too.

#7. Deliberate Decision-Making

BEST FOR: Problem-solving

Many individuals with dyslexia can see problems from all angles. They can identify the big picture and connect ideas. However, such gifted problem solvers may well have difficulty organizing a logical process to solving a problem effectively. They might overutilize their intuitive thinking and not make use of helpful information or data.

To counter that, here are seven steps for effective decision-making:

1. Define the decision by identifying a need. In other words, imagine the big picture and see what's missing.

2. Gather information, being sure to include what you already know, but also seeking new data from outside your knowledge base.

3. Identify multiple possible or alternative paths of action to achieve your decision. You can use your imagination on this step.

4. Balance the evidence. What are the pros and cons of each option? How will each of them address the need identified in step one? Evaluate the likelihood that each will achieve the goal and select a few with the best likely results.
5. Select the best alternative from those you chose in step 4. You may decide to combine a few of them.
6. Take positive action by employing the best option.
7. Evaluate the results. Has the action resolved the need? If not, you may want to restart at any point after step 1, circling through the process again.

The truth is, intuition has value as a starting point. However, a sequential action plan is a more reliable path to reaching your desired outcomes.

#8. Narrow That Big Picture

BEST FOR: **Presenting a big picture idea**

This approach will aid you in communicating your big idea, at home and at work. As big picture thinkers, we're easily misunderstood. We might have difficulty getting our message across to more detailed thinkers, who focus on all the reasons why your idea won't work.

Out-of-the-box ideas are hard to grasp for detail-oriented coworkers or family members who might need things broken down. Your ideas may seem unrealistic or might cause a disruption.

Here are some tips for communicating your ideas:

Work with a partner. To bring your idea to fruition, you will likely need someone keeping an eye on the details.

Stay on schedule. You do not want to get behind in developing your plan or get stuck working out a problem that might work itself out if you move forward. Break your planning process into steps and set reminders to keep on track (review strategy #10, "Microproductivity," in chapter 6).

Include others in your thinking. Feedback along the way will help you anticipate the objections and concerns your plan may raise. (See strategy #4, "Time to Think.")

Be an effective communicator. Realize where your team or family is coming from. Anticipate their questions. Be patient; give them time to grasp your idea. Come at your idea from different angles; use stories to make your point.

Be a good listener. Consider others' ideas. Hear what they have to say and do not get defensive when they are trying to help.

#9. Reaching the Goal

BEST FOR: Utilizing a team

You might be the u in unique, but you cannot do everything alone. Use connectiveness to form a team, whether at home for household responsibilities or at work, to share the load. A common trait among entrepreneurs is sharing their vision with a supporting team who works alongside them to reach a goal.

Determination and goal persistence may be your strengths. Avoid these potential downsides to being overly focused on an objective when incorporating other family or team members:

- Micromanaging others
- Seeming unapproachable
- Appearing insensitive to others' concerns
- Establishing yourself as irreplaceable to the job

Awareness is key. Follow these guidelines for building true teamwork:

1. Bring team and family members into the plan (strategy #8).

2. Teach others the skills they need, with patience.

3. Allow your team and family members to fail and then self-evaluate. Don't rush to save them or point out their lesson. Grit is developed through one's own experience, not someone else's.

4. Use a guided questioning approach to problems. Restrain from giving an answer too quickly. Allowing others a chance to figure things out instills ownership. You want your team or family members to feel they have an invested part of a bigger whole.

5. Have a backup plan. If it turns out your big idea is wrong, what will you do?

#10. Fun Brain Pastimes

BEST FOR: Supercharging problem-solving skills

These activities will provide some innovative ways to build on your problem-solving skills by activating the creative areas of your brain. Plus, they're an excuse to have fun!

Participate in dance. Science has shown that dancing has a positive impact on neural processing and can engage convergent thinking.

Play logic games or solve puzzles. Build up your brain power with activities like sudoku or chess.

Get high-quality sleep. Studies have shown that the rapid eye movement (REM) phase of sleep can help the brain connect random ideas. If you don't feel rested during the day, you're not sleeping enough.

Combine exercise with music. Listening to music during a workout has been shown to enhance verbal fluency.

Take part in a recreational sport. Studies have suggested playing a multitasking sport promotes brain activity.

Create mental distance. Studies have shown that when we take a step back from our thoughts, we find a solution. Try meditation, yoga, or other stress-relieving activities or hobbies.

Rely on others. When you're stuck in your thoughts, ask someone else's opinion. Take a friend to coffee.

Conclusion

Dyslexia does not need to hold you back. Embracing your strengths builds confidence, just as hard work has yielded resilience and facing adversity has nurtured empathy on your journey with dyslexia. Furthermore, being "normal" is outdated. Society is embracing mental diversity in new and exciting ways. Dyslexic skills like big picture thinking, problem-solving, understanding different perspectives, storytelling, and more are being sought after in today's workforce. Own your inherent strengths; wear them proudly.

CHAPTER 8

Dyslexia in the Real World

In this chapter, we'll close out our time together by observing how dyslexia operates in real-world scenarios. There's little doubt that adults with dyslexia face stressful, overwhelming challenges in matters of daily living. So let's explore some scenes and situations that illustrate how those challenges come up and the ways that the concepts in this book can help you navigate them.

10 Real-World Scenarios and Actionable Steps

Each of the scenarios in this chapter is independent of the others, so you can choose to read them all or skip to the ones that seem most applicable to you.

An Orton-Gillingham Story

SPEAKS TO: Improving literacy

Kathleen participated in her library's adult literacy program and was sent to me to be evaluated for dyslexia. She's bright and accomplished in her life, but she was not gaining skills in her reading.

In our initial interview, Kathleen shared, "I hide my dyslexia at my work and home. I feel I can't take on certain responsibilities. In my job, I have a lot of anxiety. I do the work, but if I have to read, I play it off. All day long, I'm on my toes so that I don't get caught off guard."

She described finally seeking help after a lifetime of secrecy. "I'm tired of dyslexia holding me back in work, school, and life," she said. "You hear about success stories. I want to be one. I would like to learn to read and write so I won't be embarrassed."

I diagnosed Kathleen with dyslexia and recommended a structured literacy program. Kathleen's tutor began training in an Orton-Gillingham curriculum.

A year later, Kathleen shares a different relationship with reading, telling me: "I recognized a lot of words just fine before. But now, when I come across a word I don't know, I can try to break it down. Words make more sense. I meet with a reading tutor twice a week. And I'm beginning to actually read."

Spelling

SPEAKS TO: Building self-confidence in writing

Nikki, a middle school teacher, reports that her most significant predicament is spelling. "Spellcheck sometimes actually makes it worse. It's embarrassing!" she exclaims.

When writing on the board in class, Nikki sometimes forgets how to spell a simple word like **necessary**. Typically, she writes it several times to see which spelling looks correct. However, that is not possible in front of critical middle schoolers.

Also, correspondence to colleagues and parents takes Nikki an exceedingly long time. She's sensitive to how her writing might appear and fears making seemingly careless errors, like forgetting a word or using the wrong word. Nikki passes everything she writes through an editing app. Even still, she finds mistakes. Nikki is losing her confidence in teaching, and self-doubt is creeping in.

Nikki might seek help from an educational therapist to isolate the type of mistakes she's making. Depending on the results, Nikki might work on:

- Breaking words into smaller parts
- Slowing down her pronunciation
- Learning tricks to recall high-frequency words

Nikki might also devise a response for when she feels trapped with a mistake in front of her class. First, she could admit to her struggle, which would also help her students be more aware and accepting of themselves and others. Second, she could ask her students for help, even reward them if they spot a mistake.

Formulating Words

SPEAKS TO: Recalling words in midlife

Mandy, a former client, is an occupational therapist in her late 40s. She expresses a growing struggle in formulating words verbally. "I have so much knowledge in my mind," she shares. "But when asked to explain, I struggle to find the right words. This has been very harmful!" Mandy has been interviewing for new jobs in hospitals and worries about giving potential employers the wrong impression.

Some new research impacting midlife women might help Mandy understand her struggle. In her latest edition of Overcoming Dyslexia, Sally Shaywitz offers an insight: Midlife women nearing menopause may experience increasing difficulty recalling words and reading because of their dyslexia. For some women, this phenomenon could begin as early as their late 30s.

To improve, Mandy might develop a personal word bank. For each interview, she could write a handful of key words on a small 3x5 card to review before her meetings or even keep in her hand.

Knowing the reason for her struggle and normalizing her mental well-being should bring Mandy a sense of calmness and more confidence. She would also benefit from casually acknowledging her loss for words during conversations. Besides, there might be other midlife women on the panel who could relate.

Mild Social Anxiety

SPEAKS TO: Building social confidence

Roberto avoids close relationships because of his dyslexia, but he misses them. As soon as he starts making friends with someone, a voice in his head echoes: "You're going to say the wrong thing," and "What if they found out?" He's felt this way since high school. Now, in his mid-20s, his anxiety has gotten worse.

Roberto tends to overthink social situations. He doesn't have the best timing in deciding when and how to tell others about his dyslexia. It's easier to not say anything. When he makes mistakes, he feels stupid. He tries to convince himself that he likes being alone. But he knows that isn't true.

Envisioning the big picture, Roberto could address the situation by leaning into his ability to plan. Roberto could start hanging out at coffee shops and public spaces where people gather, attending the same places repetitively. Eventually he might begin conversing with other regulars and feel more confident. After he grows comfortable with one-to-one interactions in this low-pressure way and at his own pace, he might consider a more intimate relationship. With the help of his counselor, he could identify appropriate ways to express his struggles with dyslexia.

A Philanthropic Support Group

SPEAKS TO: Connectiveness

Matilda, an Orton-Gillingham tutor, wants to connect colleagues who can support each other and share ideas. Matilda herself has dyslexia, and connecting people satisfies her fondness for connecting with others. Also, she spots a need in the community: The schools in her area do not know much about dyslexia. She thinks others who are working with dyslexia would want to join forces and educate the community.

New to the area, Matilda doesn't know anyone. She thinks of consulting an online directory to find others in her profession. She also decides to call some popular curriculum publishers and request contact info for certified tutors in her neighborhood.

Matilda quickly collects contact information for a handful of people. After developing a script to introduce herself and the purpose for reaching out, Matilda calls a few. She is surprised by everyone's enthusiasm. They had not thought to get together before. Many had been in the area for years, each feeling like they were practicing on an island.

The group begins meeting every month during the school year. They recognize the need to collaborate and educate their community. One group member will contact local libraries that offer free event spaces. Other members plan to take turns giving short presentations to parents, teachers, and community leaders on dyslexia at different libraries around the community. Matilda and her friends are not alone any longer, in part thanks to Matilda's gift of connectiveness.

Build It and They Will Come

SPEAKS TO: Creating a vision

Rachel is a city planner. She's trying to attract clientele from out of town. Surrounding communities have been growing, but hers has not. Their township does not offer coveted venues like a shopping mall or family fitness facility. Rachel feels that if she could highlight some aspects unique to their locality, it could bring more growth opportunities.

Instead of writing a report to explain the situation to community stakeholders, Rachel decides to use storytelling and visual elements to plan a picture of the future. She plans to commission professional photographs to update the town's website and create promotional materials. Focusing on the most unique and appealing aspects of their community, she develops a visual depiction of what resident families might enjoy in five years with economic and population growth.

Rachel plans to connect with investors like small chain stores and corporations, whose new facilities would attract visitors, bring in new families, and bring jobs, too.

She needs to share her ideas with the city council. To do this, she creates a PowerPoint that tells the story of growth for their community. Rachel feels accomplished using her gifts for connectiveness and creating a vision. The future looks promising for her township.

Planning an Event

SPEAKS TO: Prioritizing and initiating tasks to plan an event

Joe wants to plan a surprise 25th wedding anniversary party for his wife in two months. But he knows planning an event will be difficult for him. He will need to decide on a date, find a venue and a caterer, consider a guest list, and so on, all of which are the kinds of tasks his wife would typically take care of. He knows there will be many details to keep track of, like the invitations; deliveries; ordering tables, chairs, and flowers; and more. Joe isn't sure where to start, and time is running out.

His first step is to choose between:

- Securing a venue
- Hiring a caterer
- Putting together a guest list

At first it seems impossible to prioritize those three details. But stepping back and looking at the big picture, Joe realizes that the size of the guest list will determine what kind of venue is needed and that the venue may have suggestions for caterers they've worked with.

Seeing how easily he might get overwhelmed, Joe decides to ask his sister-in-law and his wife's best friend to help. Other friends have already offered to assist with decorating and setting up. Joe begins looking forward to the expression on his wife's face on their special day.

Filling Out a Job Application

SPEAKS TO: Problem-solving

Just out of high school, Hannah is looking for an entry-level job. Some applications are online; some are paper and pencil. Either way, filling out any job application seems to take Hannah forever; she lives in fear of what mistakes she will make. The job is often filled by the time Hannah feels comfortable turning in her application.

Hannah uses her problem-solving skills to plan a solution. A friend suggests that she check her local library or community center for resume workshops. Also, Hannah begins keeping a document of key phrases and bits of information that she can access on her phone or computer. When filling out online applications, she can copy and paste from that document, which has already been checked for accuracy. For paper applications, Hannah will make extra copies of the application form so she can start over if she makes a mistake.

To avoid rethinking each application, Hannah has added brief descriptions to her existing document to copy and paste into cover letters and applications. The resume process has provided Hannah with a sense of accomplishment. Now, she feels empowered in her job search. She tells herself, "I will make a valuable employee."

Improv

SPEAKS TO: Slowing down, allowing yourself the time

Glenda is an actor taking an online seminar. Her task is to role-play some improvised dramatic scenes. Glenda has always enjoyed performing on stage and is good with scripted material. But improvisation never comes easy. She wonders if that's a result of dyslexia.

Let's look at what is being tasked when creating an improv scenario. After being given a prompt to start from, you must:

- Retrieve the words that best articulate your ideas and pronounce them correctly
- Think of what the audience will need to hear for the scene to make sense
- Hear what others in the scene are saying; react to and support their ideas
- Show vulnerability; be willing to take risks by being creative in front of a live audience

You can see how improvisation takes a great deal of working memory. Unfortunately, by definition, this kind of performance cannot be prepared; it's invented on the fly. Glenda really wants to improve her improv skills, so what should she do?

Glenda can lean on a few inherent strengths by:

- Taking a few extra minutes to process the prompt and organize her thoughts
- Connecting the prompt to personal experiences in her past
- Using her problem-spotting skills to imagine a conflict from that memory
- Using her gift of global thinking to connect that conflict back to the prompt and create the scene

Because of anxiety, Glenda tends to rush. But slowing down and managing the prompt may be more helpful than rushing to come up with the "right" answer.

Accessing Your Intelligence

SPEAKS TO: Utilizing technology

Bryce must read from time to time at work. His dyslexia makes reading challenging. When he reads print, he often must read the text several times to understand it. Fortunately, the material at work is now available in digital form. Bryce downloaded a reading app to read sections of documents that he could not make out with a first pass. Bryce might also:

- Add a color overlay to his screen to help ease the strain on his eyes (an option in the accessories menu of his computer)
- Utilize annotation tools to make notes and highlight important information so he won't have to reread entire documents
- Collect data to create a web diagram depicting key takeaways from his reading
- Follow embedded links to access pictures or diagrams illustrating what he reads

Bryce enjoys the efficiency of reading digital text. The process parallels how his brain works, offering him an easier way to make connections and break down the text. Besides, he can learn new technical words, which he used to skip over. Now, he can learn and speak them with confidence, adding scope to his discussions. Digital texts help Bryce feel more intelligent.

A Final Note

Congratulations on completing this book! I trust the experience has broadened your understanding of dyslexia. And I hope you'll return to these pages whenever you need a refresher or when you want to delve into newly relevant information you previously skipped over. A guidebook isn't something you read once and put on a shelf; it's meant to be a resource to keep at hand and consult whenever you need it.

Dyslexia is a lifelong condition to be embraced, not endured. Dyslexia makes life challenging, but you are strong. With every step forward, you are closer to becoming the best you. I encourage you to explore each opportunity that whets your passion and not let dyslexia keep you from pursuing your goals.

Always believe in yourself. Reading this book has put you at an advantage: You can accept your weaknesses and, more importantly, lean on your strengths. Although we all have limitations to what we can accomplish—since I have two left feet, I will never be a professional dancer—you do not need to be limited by dyslexia. Follow what you are passionate about.

Keep these points in mind when dyslexia delivers you a down day:

If you keep moving, you get there. In general, determination and tenacity are better indicators of success than intelligence or talent. We all have our own story. But the good news is you can write your own narrative. Hold on to your goals with a firm grip, and don't let go.

Diversity is an advantage. More and more, modern society is recognizing the value of diversity. As a result, employers are pursuing your skills in the job market. Have you noticed that producers are writing television characters with dyslexia into popular series? It's cool to be you!

More resources are available than ever before. I am confident you have developed your own methods, skills, work-arounds, and options for managing dyslexia. These days, with technology increasingly the default mode of conversation, improving your literacy will broaden your skills to communicate effectively and more efficiently. Reading skills aren't set in stone; they can be developed over time with practice. And practically all print is accessible with technology.

Be patient with yourself. It will take time to incorporate new skills and build new habits. Some skills will resonate with you more than others; some will be immediately helpful, while others might benefit you over time through regular practice. Celebrate every accomplishment, no matter the size, using confidence to drive you in lifelong learning. Along the way remember that the whole must be broken down into parts for us to recognize the details—and that goes for acknowledging our own progress and incremental improvement. Although I love the forest, at times, I must attend to the trees.

It has been my pleasure to walk with you in your journey so far. I suggest you find an accessible spot for this book and revisit strategies, scenarios, and resources as you continue along on your road to understanding and managing dyslexia.

Short term memory loss

need to ~~~ write down tasks & dates

Need to create my own schedules

Slow in expressing myself

good @ numbers — Sudoku etc.

Original thinking & design

I need time doing nothing to let my mind clear.

I think by feeling

People misunderstand me — what I am — what I'm saying

Printed in Dunstable, United Kingdom